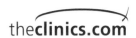

UROLOGIC CLINICS
OF NORTH AMERICA

Urologic Issues and Pregnancy

GUEST EDITOR
Deborah R. Erickson, MD

CONSULTING EDITOR
Martin I. Resnick, MD

February 2007 • Volume 34 • Number 1

SAUNDERS

An Imprint of Elsevier, Inc.
PHILADELPHIA   LONDON   TORONTO   MONTREAL   SYDNEY   TOKYO

W.B. SAUNDERS COMPANY
A Division of Elsevier Inc.

1600 John F. Kennedy Boulevard • Suite 1800 • Philadelphia, Pennsylvania 19103-2899

http://www.theclinics.com

UROLOGIC CLINICS OF NORTH AMERICA　　　　　　　Volume 34, Number 1
February 2007　　　　　　　　　　　　　　　　　　　　　ISSN 0094-0143
Editor: Kerry Holland　　　　　　　　　　　　　　ISBN-13: 978-1-4160-4824-4
　　　　　　　　　　　　　　　　　　　　　　　　　　ISBN-10: 1-4160-4824-3

The ideas and opinions expressed in *Urologic Clinics of North America* do not necessarily reflect those of the Publisher. The Publisher does not assume any responsibility for any injury and/or damage to persons or property arising out of or related to any use of the material contained in this periodical. The reader is advised to check the appropriate medical literature and the product information currently provided by the manufacturer of each drug to be administered to verify the dosage, the method and duration of administration, or contraindications. It is the responsibility of the treating physician or other health care professional, relying on independent experience and knowledge of the patient, to determine drug dosages and the best treatment for the patient. Mention of any product in this issue should not be construed as endorsement by the contributors, editors, or the Publisher of the product or manufacturers' claims.

Urologic Clinics of North America (ISSN 0094-0143) is published quarterly by Elsevier Inc., 360 Park Avenue South, New York, NY 10010-1710. Months of issue are February, May, August, and November. Business and Editorial Offices: 1600 John F. Kennedy Blvd., Suite 1800, Philadelphia, PA 19103-2899. Customer Service Office: 6277 Sea Harbor Drive, Orlando, FL 32887-4800. Periodicals postage paid at New York, NY and additional mailing offices. Subscription prices are $231.00 per year (US individuals), $358.00 per year (US institutions), $264.00 per year (Canadian individuals), $429.00 per year (Canadian institutions), $308.00 per year (foreign individuals), and $429.00 per year (foreign institutions). Foreign air speed delivery is included in all *Clinics* subscription prices. All prices are subject to change without notice. **POSTMASTER:** Send address changes to *Urologic Clinics of North America*, Elsevier Periodicals Customer Service, 6277 Sea Harbor Drive, Orlando, FL 32887-4800. **Customer Service: 1-800-654-2452 (US). From outside the US, call 1-407-345-4000.**

Urologic Clinics of North America is covered in *Index Medicus*, *Excerpta Medica*, *Current Contents/Clinical Medicine, Science Citation Index*, and *ISI/BIOMED*.

Printed in the United States of America.

GOAL STATEMENT
The goal of *Urologic Clinics of North America* is to keep practicing urologists and urology residents up to date with current clinical practice in urology by providing timely articles reviewing the state of the art in patient care.

ACCREDITATION
The *Urologic Clinics of North America* is planned and implemented in accordance with the Essential Areas and Policies of the Accreditation Council for Continuing Medical Education (ACCME) through the joint sponsorship of the University of Virginia School of Medicine and Elsevier. The University of Virginia School of Medicine is accredited by the ACCME to provide continuing medical education for physicians.

The University of Virginia School of Medicine designates this educational activity for a maximum of *15 AMA PRA Category 1 Credits™*. Physicians should only claim credit commensurate with the extent of their participation in the activity.

The American Medical Association has determined that physicians not licensed in the US who participate in this CME activity are eligible for *15 AMA PRA Category 1 Credits™*.

Credit can be earned by reading the text material, taking the CME examination online at http://www.theclinics.com/home/cme, and completing the evaluation. After taking the test, you will be required to review any and all incorrect answers. Following completion of the test and evaluation, your credit will be awarded and you may print your certificate.

FACULTY DISCLOSURE/CONFLICT OF INTEREST
The University of Virginia School of Medicine, as an ACCME accredited provider, endorses and strives to comply with the Accreditation Council for Continuing Medical Education (ACCME) Standards of Commercial Support, Commonwealth of Virginia statutes, University of Virginia policies and procedures, and associated federal and private regulations and guidelines on the need for disclosure and monitoring of proprietary and financial interests that may affect the scientific integrity and balance of content delivered in continuing medical education activities under our auspices.

The University of Virginia School of Medicine requires that all CME activities accredited through this institution be developed independently and be scientifically rigorous, balanced and objective in the presentation/discussion of its content, theories and practices.

All authors/editors participating in an accredited CME activity are expected to disclose to the readers relevant financial relationships with commercial entities occurring within the past 12 months (such as grants or research support, employee, consultant, stock holder, member of speakers bureau, etc.). The University of Virginia School of Medicine will employ appropriate mechanisms to resolve potential conflicts of interest to maintain the standards of fair and balanced education to the reader. Questions about specific strategies can be directed to the Office of Continuing Medical Education, University of Virginia School of Medicine, Charlottesville, Virginia.

The authors/editors listed below have identified no professional or financial affiliations for themselves or their spouse/partner:
Deborah R. Erickson, MD (Guest Editor); Facundo Garcia-Bournissen, MD; Scott Graziano, MD; Richard Hautmann, MD; Kerry Holland (Acquisitions Editor); Katherine C. Hubert, MD; Arundhathi Jeyabalan, MD, MSCR; Gideon Koren, MD; Chad Lagrange, MD; Kristine Y. Lain, MD, MSCR; Larry L. Leeman, MD; Kevin R. Loughlin, MD; Amanda Macejko, MD; Francis M. Martin, MD; Vernon M. Pais, Jr., MD; Jeffrey Palmer, MD, FACS, FAAP; Alice L. Payton, MD; Kathleen J. Propert, ScD; Randall Rowland, MD, PhD; Alon Shrim, MD; and, Bjoern G. Volkmer, MD.

The authors/editors listed below identified the following professional or financial affiliations for themselves or their spouse/partner:
Mary P. FitzGerald, MD is an independent contractor for Pfizer and Allergan; and is on the speaker's bureau for Medtronic.
Rebecca G. Rogers, MD is a consultant for and receives a research grant from Pfizer; and receives a research grant from Wyeth.
Anthony J. Schaeffer, MD is a consultant for Depomed, Inc., Synermed Communications, Schwarz Biosciences, and Bayer; and is on the Advisory Board for McNeil Consumer and Specialty Pharmacy and Ortho McNeil Pharmaceuticals.

Disclosure of Discussion of non-FDA approved uses for pharmaceutical products and/or medical devices:
The University of Virginia School of Medicine, as an ACCME provider, requires that all faculty presenters identify and disclose any "off label" uses for pharmaceutical and medical device products. The University of Virginia School of Medicine recommends that each physician fully review all the available data on new products or procedures prior to instituting them with patients.

TO ENROLL
To enroll in the Urologic Clinics of North America Continuing Medical Education program, call customer service at 1-800-654-2452 or visit us online at www.theclinics.com/home/cme. The CME program is available to subscribers for an additional fee of $195.00.

CONSULTING EDITOR

MARTIN I. RESNICK, MD, Lester Persky Professor and Chairman, Department of Urology, Case Medical Center, Cleveland, Ohio

GUEST EDITOR

DEBORAH R. ERICKSON, MD, Professor of Surgery, Division of Urology, Department of Surgery, University of Kentucky College of Medicine, University of Kentucky Chandler Medical Center, Lexington, Kentucky

CONTRIBUTORS

DEBORAH R. ERICKSON, MD, Professor of Surgery, Division of Urology, Department of Surgery, University of Kentucky College of Medicine, University of Kentucky Chandler Medical Center, Lexington, Kentucky

MARY P. FITZGERALD, MD, Associate Professor, Division of Female Pelvic Medicine and Reconstructive Surgery, Departments of Urology and Obstetrics/Gynecology, Loyola University Medical Center, Maywood, Illinois

FACUNDO GARCIA-BOURNISSEN, MD, Clinical Fellow, The Motherisk Program, Division of Clinical Pharmacology/Toxicology, Hospital for Sick Children, The University of Toronto, Toronto, Ontario, Canada

SCOTT GRAZIANO, MD, Assistant Professor, Department of Obstetrics/Gynecology, Loyola University Medical Center, Maywood, Illinois

RICHARD E. HAUTMANN, MD, Head, Department of Urology, University of Ulm, Ulm, Germany

KATHERINE C. HUBERT, MD, Case Western Reserve University, Cleveland, Ohio

ARUNDHATHI JEYABALAN, MD, Assistant Professor, Department of Obstetrics, Gynecology, and Reproductive Sciences, University of Pittsburgh School of Medicine, Pittsburgh, Pennsylvania

GIDEON KOREN, MD, Professor and Director, The Motherisk Program, University of Toronto, Toronto, Ontario, Canada; and Ivey Chair in Molecular Toxicology, University of Western Ontario, London, Ontario, Canada

CHAD A. LAGRANGE, MD, Endourology Fellow, Division of Urology, Department of Surgery, University of Kentucky College of Medicine, University of Kentucky Chandler Medical Center, Lexington, Kentucky

KRISTINE Y. LAIN, MD, Assistant Professor, Department of Obstetrics and Gynecology, University of Kentucky College of Medicine, University of Kentucky Chandler Medical Center, Lexington, Kentucky

LARRY L. LEEMAN, MD, Associate Professor, Department of Family and Community Medicine; and Associate Professor, Department of Obstetrics and Gynecology, University of New Mexico Health Sciences Center, Albuquerque, New Mexico

KEVIN R. LOUGHLIN, MD, Division of Urology, Brigham and Women's Hospital, Boston, Massachusetts; and Harvard Medical School, Boston, Massachusetts

AMANDA M. MACEJKO, MD, Resident, Department of Urology, Northwestern University, Chicago, Illinois

FRANCES M. MARTIN, MD, Resident, Division of Urology, Department of Surgery, University of Kentucky College of Medicine, University of Kentucky Chandler Medical Center, Lexington, Kentucky

VERNON M. PAIS JR, MD, Assistant Professor of Surgery, Division of Urology, Department of Surgery, University of Kentucky College of Medicine, University of Kentucky Chandler Medical Center, Lexington, Kentucky

JEFFREY S. PALMER, MD, FACS, FAAP, Director of Minimally Invasive Pediatric Urology, Glickman Urological Institute, Children's Hospital at Cleveland Clinic; and Assistant Professor of Surgery, Lerner College of Medicine of Case Western Reserve University, Cleveland, Ohio

ALICE L. PAYTON, MD, Resident, Division of Urology, Department of Surgery, University of Kentucky College of Medicine, University of Kentucky Chandler Medical Center, Lexington, Kentucky

KATHLEEN J. PROPERT, ScD, Associate Professor of Biostatistics, Department of Biostatistics and Epidemiology, University of Pennsylvania School of Medicine, Philadelphia, Pennsylvania

REBECCA G. ROGERS, MD, Director, Division of Urogynecology; and Associate Professor, Department of Obstetrics and Gynecology, University of New Mexico Health Sciences Center, Albuquerque, New Mexico

RANDALL G. ROWLAND, MD, PhD, Professor and Chief, Division of Urology, Department of Surgery, University of Kentucky College of Medicine, University of Kentucky Chandler Medical Center, Lexington, Kentucky

ANTHONY J. SCHAEFFER, MD, Chairman, Department of Urology, Northwestern University, Chicago, Illinois

ALON SHRIM, MD, Clinical Fellow, The Motherisk Program, Division of Clinical Pharmacology/Toxicology, Hospital for Sick Children, The University of Toronto, Toronto, Ontario, Canada

BJOERN G. VOLKMER, MD, Department of Urology, University of Ulm, Ulm, Germany

CONTENTS

aim to describe genitourinary postpartum pelvic floor changes, and review the literature regarding the impact of pregnancy or childbirth on these changes. Data is needed that compare the effects of pregnancy alone, cesarean delivery (labored and unlabored), and vaginal birth, so that physicians can better advise patients about the postpartum genitourinary tract changes they might expect.

Urologic Radiology During Pregnancy

Kevin R. Loughlin

The pregnant patient presents a unique diagnostic challenge to the urologist because the well-being of both the mother and fetus must be considered. Radiation exposure to the fetus during gestation presents risks such as cell death and teratogenic effects, carcinogenesis, and genetic effects, which must be considered when selecting diagnostic tests. However, with the exercise of good clinical judgment and the use of the armamentarium of diagnostic imaging modalities available, the pregnant patient can be managed with minimal, if any, radiation exposure to the fetus.

Pharmaceutical Agents and Pregnancy in Urology Practice

Alon Shrim, Facundo Garcia-Bournissen, and Gideon Koren

Urologic medical conditions are not frequently encountered during pregnancy. Still, urologists often are asked to treat pregnant patients for conditions that require prescriptions. In the generally healthy population of pregnant women, the use of pharmaceutical agents is usually reserved for women who have either infections or necessary surgical procedures. This article addresses the implications for pregnancy of common urologic conditions in generally healthy pregnant women, namely simple urinary tract infections that demand nitrofurantoin and complex urinary tract infections that necessitate fluoroquinolones treatment. It also examines the implications of nonobstetric surgical intervention.

Asymptomatic Bacteriuria and Symptomatic Urinary Tract Infections During Pregnancy

Amanda M. Macejko and Anthony J. Schaeffer

Urinary tract infections are common complications of pregnancy; upper tract infections in particular may lead to significant morbidity for both the mother and fetus. Bacteriuria is a significant risk factor for developing pyelonephritis in pregnant women. Therefore, proper screening and treatment of bacteriuria during pregnancy is necessary to prevent complications. All women should be screened for bacteriuria in the first trimester, and women with a history of recurrent urinary tract infections or anomalies should have repeat bacteriuria screening throughout pregnancy. Treatment of bacteriuria should include 3-day therapy with appropriate antimicrobials, and women should be followed closely after treatment because recurrence may occur in up to one third of patients.

Urolithiasis in Pregnancy

Vernon M. Pais Jr, Alice L. Payton, and Chad A. LaGrange

The presentation of urolithiasis is often dramatic, but rarely is it more anxiety provoking than during pregnancy. The evaluation and the intervention are often approached with trepidation as the health of the mother and the fetus must be taken into account. The typical diagnostic course and surgical management used in the nonpregnant population must be reevaluated in the expectant mother. Failure to promptly diagnose and manage urolithiasis during pregnancy may have adverse consequences for mother and child. The authors present a review of the relevant anatomic and physiologic changes of pregnancy as they affect stone disease and outline options for radiologic evaluation and surgical management.

CONTENTS

FORTHCOMING ISSUES

RECENT ISSUES

THE CLINICS ARE NOW AVAILABLE ONLINE!

Access your subscription at:
http://www.theclinics.com

**UROLOGIC
CLINICS
of North America**

Urol Clin N Am 34 (2007) xi

Foreword

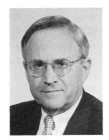

Martin I. Resnick, MD
Consulting Editor

I have no doubt that this issue of the *Urologic Clinics of North America*, addressing urologic problems associated with pregnancy, will be of great interest, not only to urologists but also to other physicians caring for the pregnant patient. Though fortunately, most pregnancies proceed with little or no problems, complications do occur, and a significant number of these are associated with the urinary tract.

Dr. Erickson has assembled an excellent list of pertinent topics and appropriate authors to address the many issues associated with this topic. In addition to reviewing recognized changes in the upper and lower urinary tract associated with pregnancy, varied problems and complications are discussed. Some are common, such as urinary tract infection and urolithiasis, but others, including urologic malignancies and specific issues related to urinary diversion, fortunately occur uncommonly.

All should find this issue of the *Urologic Clinics of North America* of value. I believe it will be used as a frequent reference for those caring for these patients.

Martin I. Resnick, MD
Department of Urology
Case Medical Center
Cleveland, OH, USA

E-mail address: martin.resnick@case.edu

UROLOGIC
CLINICS
of North America

Preface

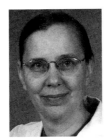

Deborah R. Erickson, MD
Guest Editor

Going through previous issues of the *Urologic Clinics of North America*, we occasionally see articles about specific urologic problems in pregnancy. However, this is the first issue completely dedicated to pregnancy. Being the guest editor was a great pleasure, especially having the opportunity to identify and work with a fine group of authors from various specialty areas. This timely and relevant issue provides state-of-the-art information from experts in their respective fields.

The article topics include the effects of pregnancy and delivery on the genitourinary tract, with separate articles on upper tract changes during pregnancy, lower tract changes during pregnancy, and postpartum changes. Also, as we all know, pregnant women are not immune from urologic disease, but their evaluation and management may be changed. Some articles discuss topics with many applications, such as urologic radiology and use of pharmaceutical agents during pregnancy. Other articles focus on managing specific urologic problems during pregnancy: infections, stones, malignancies, and interstitial cystitis. Also, with modern medical care, previously rare urologic scenarios are now frequent, including fetal urologic anomalies and pregnancy in women with urinary diversions.

In some cases, different authors had different opinions about specific urologic issues during pregnancy. Such controversies are not unusual; physicians often have to make decisions with an incomplete knowledge base. In pregnancy it is especially important to evaluate risks and benefits to both mother and fetus, combining astute clinical judgment with the patient's informed choices.

This issue of the *Urologic Clinics of North America* will be an important reference for urologists and other clinicians who care for women of childbearing age. I am very grateful to all of the authors for their valuable contributions and to the editorial staff at Elsevier, Inc. for their expert assistance.

Deborah R. Erickson, MD
Division of Urology, Department of Surgery
University of Kentucky College of Medicine
University of Kentucky Chandler Medical Center
800 Rose Street, Room MS-269
Lexington, KY 40536-0298, USA

E-mail address: Dreric2@email.uky.edu

doi:10.1016/j.ucl.2006.10.012

ELSEVIER
SAUNDERS

Urol Clin N Am 34 (2007) 1–6

UROLOGIC
CLINICS
of North America

Anatomic and Functional Changes of the Upper Urinary Tract During Pregnancy

Arundhathi Jeyabalan, MD[a],*, Kristine Y. Lain, MD[b]

[a]Division of Maternal-Fetal Medicine, Department of Obstetrics, Gynecology, and Reproductive Sciences,
University of Pittsburgh School of Medicine, Magee-Womens Hospital, Room 2225, 300 Halket Street,
Pittsburgh, PA 15206, USA
[b]Division of Maternal-Fetal Medicine, Department of Obstetrics and Gynecology,
University of Kentucky College of Medicine, University of Kentucky Chandler Medical Center,
800 Rose Street, Room C-365, Lexington, KY 40536-0293, USA

An appreciation of the maternal physiologic adaptations that occur in the renal system during pregnancy is fundamental to the understanding and proper clinical management of normal pregnancy, renal disorders in the gravid patient, and pregnancy-specific conditions such as pre-eclampsia. In this article, we will first address the anatomic changes that occur in the upper urinary tract in normal pregnancy, followed by the dramatic alterations in maternal renal hemodynamics and glomerular filtration. We will also briefly discuss renal handling of various substrates in pregnancy, including protein, uric acid, and glucose. Finally, the direct relevance of these changes to the clinician caring for pregnant women will be summarized.

Anatomic changes in the upper urinary tract

The upper urinary tract undergoes a variety of anatomic changes during normal pregnancy. Secondary to changes in total vascular volume, renal vascular volume and interstitial volume increase. As a result, overall kidney dimensions increase by approximately 1 cm, and renal volume increases by as much as 30% [1,2].

In addition to volume increases, there is dilation of the collecting system, including the renal calyces, pelvis, and ureters, leading to a physiologic hydronephrosis and hydroureter that occur in 80% of women by midpregnancy [3]. Ureteral dilation occurs to some degree in the majority of patients, most commonly on the right side, and is often greater on the right side than on the left [4]. The cause of dilation is most likely secondary to mechanical compression from an enlarging uterus and ovarian vein plexus [3]. Dilation is rarely present below the pelvic brim [4]. The effect of progesterone and hence the contribution of hormones to these changes is unclear. Marchant [5] suggested that progesterone may influence smooth muscle relaxation, but other investigators have demonstrated no correlation between degree of dilatation and progesterone or estradiol concentrations [6].

Renal hemodynamics and glomerular filtration rate during normal pregnancy

Both *glomerular filtration rate* (GFR) and *renal plasma flow* (RPF) increase markedly in normal pregnancy. In a detailed compilation of rigorously selected studies, GFR and effective RPF were increased by 40% to 65% and 50% to 85%, respectively, in the first half of gestation (Fig. 1) [7]. These studies are particularly noteworthy because (1) GFR and RPF were measured using the "gold standard" (renal clearances of inulin and para-aminohippurate), (2) GFR and RPF in the first half of gestation were compared with

---

* Corresponding author.

E-mail address: ajeyabalan@mail.magee.edu
(A. Jeyabalan).

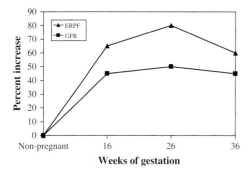

Fig. 1. GFR and effective renal plasma flow (ERPF) during pregnancy. Renal plasma flow increases most dramatically in the first trimester, then reaches peak levels 50% to 80% above baseline nonpregnant levels by the beginning of the third trimester, with a subsequent decline in the latter part of pregnancy toward term. GFR, which is largely determined by RPF, follows a similar pattern of increase, by about 50% with more of a plateau at term. (*Data from* Conrad KP, Lindheimer MD. Renal and cardiovascular alterations. In: Lindheimer MD, Roberts JM, Cunningham FG, editors. Chesley's hypertensive disorders in pregnancy. 2nd edition. Stamford (CT): Appleton and Lange; 1999. p. 263–326.)

Table 1
Normal laboratory variables in pregnancy

Variable	Normal value in pregnancy
Creatinine	0.5 mg/dL
Blood urea nitrogen (BUN)	9.0 mg/dL
Glomerular filtration rate	$\uparrow$ ~40%–65% above baseline
Creatinine clearance	$\uparrow$ ~25% above baseline
Uric acid	2.0–3.0 mg/dL
Urinary protein excretion	<300 mg/24 h
Urinary albumin excretion	<20 mg/24 h
Sodium retention over pregnancy	900–950 mmol
Plasma osmolality	$\downarrow$ ~10 mOsm/kg H_2O
Pco_2	$\downarrow$ ~10 mm Hg below baseline
Serum bicarbonate	18–20 mEq/L
Urinary glucose excretion	Variable

pre-pregnant or postpartum values, and (3) urinary tract dead space was minimized [7]. As noted earlier, RPF rises to a greater degree than GFR, resulting in a reduced filtration fraction (filtration fraction= GFR/RPF). Toward the end of pregnancy, RPF declines while GFR is maintained.

Creatinine clearance, as determined by a 24-hour urine collection, is used clinically to assess renal function and estimate GFR. Although endogenous creatinine is both filtered by the glomerulus and secreted by the proximal tubule of the kidney, creatinine clearance is a reliable measure of GFR during pregnancy [7,8]. The exception is in situations such as renal disease where GFR is markedly reduced, and creatinine clearance may overestimate the actual GFR. Creatinine clearance increases moderately during pregnancy and ranges from 100 to 150 mL per minute (Table 1). The 24-hour urine collection technique to determine creatinine clearance and estimate GFR has been used to demonstrate that the GFR changes occur quite early in gestation. Davison and Noble [9] demonstrated that GFR rises 25% by the fourth week of pregnancy (from last menstrual period) and 45% by 9 weeks' gestation. In fact, these renal hemodynamic alterations are among the earliest and most dramatic maternal adaptations to pregnancy.

Serum creatinine and *urea*, commonly used markers for renal function, are both reduced during pregnancy as a result of the elevated GFR. Average values for serum creatinine and urea are 0.5 mg/dL and 9.0 mg/dL, respectively, compared with nonpregnant values of 0.8 mg/dL and 13.0 mg/dL [7]. Circulating creatinine levels are determined primarily by skeletal muscle production and urinary excretion, with relatively free filtration of creatinine across the glomerular barrier. In pregnancy, skeletal muscle production of creatinine remains relatively constant while GFR is markedly increased, resulting in reduced levels of circulating creatinine. Urea is also freely filtered at the level of the glomerulus. The renal handling of urea during pregnancy is complex and is discussed in more detail later (see "Renal handling of uric acid in pregnancy").

Mechanisms of renal hemodynamic alterations in pregnancy

The precise mechanisms underlying the gestational renal hemodynamic alterations remain incompletely understood. Reduced renal vascular resistance is ultimately responsible for the increased renal blood flow and therefore for the increased GFR. These early alterations occur in anticipation of the future needs of the fetal-placental unit and may even precede the early gestational changes in plasma volume and cardiac output [10,11].

Animal models have been useful in studying the renal adaptations to pregnancy. The gravid rat model has been used because it demonstrates renal, cardiovascular, and endocrine changes comparable to human pregnancy. Baylis and colleagues [12,13] have applied the micropuncture technique in Munich-Wistar rats at midgestation when renal hemodynamic changes are maximal. These investigators demonstrated that the increase in GFR at the level of the individual nephron is due to a rise in plasma flow with no associated increase in glomerular hydrostatic pressure. Concomitant decreases in both preglomerular and postglomerular arteriolar resistances in the pregnant rat result in these renal adaptations. Although it is not feasible to perform such studies on pregnant women, indirect evidence using membrane modeling to study the filtration barrier in pregnancy supports these animal findings [14,15]. Pregnancy-induced renal hemodynamic alterations and their underlying mechanisms have also been studied extensively by Conrad and others [8,10,16] using the chronically instrumented, conscious gravid rat model.

Hormones have been implicated in these early renal hemodynamic alterations. Interestingly, GFR and RPF rise during the luteal phase of the menstrual cycle even before pregnancy is achieved. GFR increases by 20% in the second half of the menstrual cycle [9], with a further rise to 40% to 65% above baseline values in the early part of gestation. These findings support the hypothesis that maternal ovarian hormones or pregnancy hormones produced by the fetal-placental unit may be important in effecting these gestational alterations in the renal system.

Numerous hormonal changes occur during pregnancy, and many of these have been studied in the context of renal and cardiovascular alterations. The role of the sex steroid hormones, estrogen and progesterone, has been studied [7]. Estrogen does not appear to influence RPF or GFR, although it certainly has a role in increasing blood flow to other reproductive and nonreproductive organs [17,18]. By contrast, administration of progesterone in human and animal studies resulted in an increase in RPF and GFR, but to a much lesser degree than is observed in pregnancy [19,20]. Further study is needed to determine the precise role of progesterone and its metabolites in the pregnancy-induced renal hemodynamic changes. Peptide hormones of maternal

and placental origin have also been investigated in this regard. The role of prolactin remains controversial [21], and placental lactogens have not been investigated. Relaxin, which arises from the corpus luteum of the ovary in both rats and women, has been studied extensively using the rat model [8]. Conrad and colleagues [22] have demonstrated that GFR and effective RPF changes comparable to those of midgestation are observed when recombinant human relaxin or porcine relaxin is administered to conscious, chronically instrumented female nonpregnant rats. These changes were also observed in ovariectomized female rats [23], and even in male rats administered relaxin [24]. Furthermore, administration of relaxin-neutralizing antibodies to midterm pregnant rats abolished the increase in GFR and RPF [23].

Extensive work has demonstrated that the pregnancy- and relaxin-induced renal vasodilatation and hyperfiltration occur via an endothelial endothelin-B receptor and nitric oxide pathway [24–26]. Recently, vascular gelatinase or gelatinases, specifically matrix metalloproteinase-2, were shown to be a necessary component of this renal vasodilatory pathway [27]. Although human studies are limited, there is some evidence that relaxin may have an important role in the renal hemodynamic changes of pregnancy. In women who lack ovarian function with undetectable serum relaxin levels and achieve pregnancy through egg donation, the gestational increase in GFR is less than that seen in women who have normal ovarian function [28]. When recombinant human relaxin was administered for a short period to healthy volunteers, it resulted in an increase in RPF by 60%, without an increase in GFR [29]. Chronic administration of relaxin in the context of a scleroderma treatment trial also resulted in an increase in creatinine clearance by 15% to 20% above predicted levels [30]. Although not definitive, these findings in human and animal studies suggest an important role for relaxin in the early and dramatic renal adaptations that occur in pregnancy.

Renal handling of substrates in normal pregnancy

Uric acid

Serum uric acid levels are decreased by 25% to 35% in normal pregnancy, with a nadir of 2 to 3 mg/dL at 24 weeks' gestation and levels increasing toward nonpregnant values in the third trimester

[7,31]. The primary sources of uric acid include purine breakdown and dietary intake, and its clearance is primarily by renal excretion. Approximately 95% of circulating acid is unbound and undergoes glomerular filtration. Uric acid also undergoes proximal tubular reabsorption and secretion. In humans, net uric acid reabsorption occurs, with only 7% to 12% of the filtered load undergoing urinary excretion (reviewed in [7]). Although multiple factors can play a role in circulating uric acid alterations in pregnancy, altered renal handling is most likely the major contributing factor. The mechanism for increased uric acid clearance by the kidney during gestation is increased GFR, reduced proximal tubular reabsorption, or both [31,32].

Conditions that lead to plasma volume contraction, such as pre-eclampsia, can lead to decreased uric acid clearance and increased circulating levels. Uric acid has garnered considerable attention in the prediction, diagnosis, and pathophysiology of pre-eclampsia [7,33–37].

Protein

Assessment of urinary protein excretion is important in the detection and monitoring of renal disease, as well as of pathologic conditions specific to pregnancy, such as pre-eclampsia. During pregnancy, both total protein excretion and urinary albumin excretion are increased compared with nonpregnant levels, particularly after 20 weeks' gestation [7]. Based on the results of a longitudinal study evaluating women before conception, through pregnancy, and post partum, as well as on smaller cross-sectional studies, the average 24-hour total protein and albumin excretion are 200 mg and 12 mg, respectively, with upper limits of 300 mg per 24 hours and 20 mg per 24 hours [38–40].

In addition, low-molecular-weight proteins and renal tubular enzymes are increased in pregnancy, implicating reduced proximal tubular resorptive capacity [7,41]. Increased GFR and possible alterations in the glomerular charge selectivity also contribute to the gestational proteinuria and albuminuria. No apparent change occurs in glomerular permselectivity based on molecular weight or size during normal pregnancy.

Sodium and volume homeostasis

During normal pregnancy, systemic vascular resistance is markedly reduced, with associated increases in plasma volume and cardiac output

[7,42]. This gradual expansion in plasma volume is achieved by net sodium retention of 900 to 950 mEq over the course of pregnancy. The net reabsorption of sodium by the renal tubule despite the large filtered load is a remarkable adaptation of the renal tubule in pregnancy.

A physiologic decrease in plasma osmolality also occurs beginning in early gestation, reaching a nadir around the 10th week and remaining stable for the duration of pregnancy. This finding has been attributed to a "resetting of the osmostat," with an appropriate vasopressin response around an altered threshold.

Acid-base homeostasis

The kidney also plays an important role in acid-base homeostasis. The primary acid-base alteration of pregnancy results from an increase in minute ventilation, which causes a relative respiratory alkalosis. A compensatory response occurs in the kidney, with increased bicarbonate excretion and a decline in serum bicarbonate levels. This decrease in serum bicarbonate may limit the buffering capacity in pregnancy.

Glucose

Glucose is freely filtered and almost completely reabsorbed by a sodium-coupled active transport in the proximal tubule. A small amount of glucose is also absorbed in the collecting tubule. In nonpregnancy, minimal glucose (<125 mg/d) is excreted in the urine [43]. Generally, glucose in the urine does not appear until the plasma concentrations exceed the maximal tubular capacity for reabsorption or a threshold concentration of 200 to 240 mg/dL [43]. Renal glucosuria is asymptomatic, occurring when variable amounts of glucose are excreted despite normal serum concentrations, and is indicative of a tubular abnormality [44].

In pregnancy, an increase in plasma volume results in both an increased GFR and an increased tubular flow rate. This increased flow rate may limit the ability of the proximal tubule to completely reabsorb glucose, resulting in a physiologic glucosuria of pregnancy [44]. Davison and colleagues [45] demonstrated less effective reabsorption of glucose during pregnancy, with return to normal post partum, in 29 otherwise healthy women. In addition, animal studies have suggested that the glucose resorption in the distal nephron may be decreased [46]. Therefore, the increase in excreted glucose in late pregnancy may be secondary to decreased efficiency of both the proximal tubule and the collecting tubule. Overall, the amount of excreted glucose in the third trimester is increased several-fold compared with the small amount excreted by nonpregnant individuals. Because of these changes in renal handling of glucose and the normal appearance of glucose in the urine, the use of glucosuria as a screen for pregnancy-related glucose intolerance is not particularly helpful.

Summary

Numerous changes occur in the renal system during normal pregnancy. These can affect normal laboratory parameters and are important to understand when one is caring for the gravid patient. The authors have provided a quick reference table with normal pregnancy values for a number of relevant laboratory parameters that are altered during pregnancy (see Table 1).

References

[1] Bailey RR, Rolleston GL. Kidney length and ureteric dilatation in the puerperium. J Obstet Gynaecol Br Commonw 1971;78:55–61.

[2] Christensen T, Klebe JG, Bertelsen V, et al. Changes in renal volume during normal pregnancy. Acta Obstet Gynecol Scand 1989;68:541–3.

[3] Rasmussen PE, Nielsen FR. Hydronephrosis during pregnancy: a literature survey. Eur J Obstet Gynecol Reprod Biol 1988;27:249–59.

[4] Schulman A, Herlinger H. Urinary tract dilatation in pregnancy. Br J Radiol 1975;48:638–45.

[5] Marchant DJ. Effects of pregnancy and progestational agents on the urinary tract. Am J Obstet Gynecol 1972;112:487–501.

[6] Au KK, Woo JS, Tang LC, et al. Aetiological factors in the genesis of pregnancy hydronephrosis. Aust N Z J Obstet Gynaecol 1985;25:248–51.

[7] Conrad KP, Lindheimer MD. Renal and cardiovascular alterations. In: Lindheimer MD, Roberts JM, Cunningham FG, editors. Chesley's hypertensive disorders in pregnancy. 2nd edition. Stamford (CT): Appleton and Lange; 1999. p. 263–326.

[8] Conrad KP, Novak J, Danielson LA, et al. Mechanisms of renal vasodilation and hyperfiltration during pregnancy: current perspectives and potential implications for preeclampsia. Endothelium 2005; 12:57–62.

[9] Davison JM, Noble MC. Serial changes in 24 hour creatinine clearance during normal menstrual cycles and the first trimester of pregnancy. Br J Obstet Gynaecol 1981;88:10–7.

[10] Conrad KP. Mechanisms of renal vasodilation and hyperfiltration during pregnancy. J Soc Gynecol Investig 2004;11:438–48.

[11] Lindheimer MD, Davison JM, Katz AI. The kidney and hypertension in pregnancy: twenty exciting years. Semin Nephrol 2001;21:173–89.

[12] Baylis C. Glomerular filtration rate in normal and abnormal pregnancies. Semin Nephrol 1999;19: 133–9.

[13] Baylis C. The mechanism of the increase in glomerular filtration rate in the twelve-day pregnant rat. J Physiol 1980;305:405–14.

[14] Roberts M, Lindheimer MD, Davison JM. Altered glomerular permselectivity to neutral dextrans and heteroporous membrane modeling in human pregnancy. Am J Physiol 1996;270:F338–43.

[15] Moran P, Baylis PH, Lindheimer MD, et al. Glomerular ultrafiltration in normal and preeclamptic pregnancy. J Am Soc Nephrol 2003;14:648–52.

[16] Conrad KP. Renal hemodynamics during pregnancy in chronically catheterized, conscious rats. Kidney Int 1984;26:24–9.

[17] Magness RR, Phernetton TM, Zheng J. Systemic and uterine blood flow distribution during prolonged infusion of 17beta-estradiol. Am J Physiol 1998;275:H731–43.

[18] Christy NP, Shaver JC. Estrogens and the kidney. Kidney Int 1974;6:366–76.

[19] Oparil S, Ehrlich EN, Lindheimer MD. Effect of progesterone on renal sodium handling in man: relation to aldosterone excretion and plasma renin activity. Clin Sci Mol Med 1975;49:139–47.

[20] Omer S, Mulay S, Cernacek P, et al. Attenuation of renal effects of atrial natriuretic factor during rat pregnancy. Am J Physiol 1995;268:F416–22.

[21] Conrad KP. Possible mechanisms for changes in renal hemodynamics during pregnancy: studies from animal models. Am J Kidney Dis 1987;9:253–9.

[22] Danielson LA, Sherwood OD, Conrad KP. Relaxin is a potent renal vasodilator in conscious rats. J Clin Invest 1999;103:525–33.

[23] Novak J, Danielson LA, Kerchner LJ, et al. Relaxin is essential for renal vasodilation during pregnancy in conscious rats. J Clin Invest 2001;107:1469–75.

[24] Danielson LA, Kercher LJ, Conrad KP. Impact of gender and endothelin on renal vasodilation and hyperfiltration induced by relaxin in conscious rats. Am J Physiol Regul Integr Comp Physiol 2000; 279:R1298–304.

[25] Conrad KP, Gandley RE, Ogawa T, et al. Endothelin mediates renal vasodilation and hyperfiltration during pregnancy in chronically instrumented conscious rats. Am J Physiol 1999;276: F767–76.

[26] Danielson LA, Conrad KP. Acute blockade of nitric oxide synthase inhibits renal vasodilation and hyperfiltration during pregnancy in chronically instrumented conscious rats. J Clin Invest 1995;96: 482–90.

[27] Jeyabalan A, Novak J, Danielson LA, et al. Essential role for vascular gelatinase activity in relaxin-induced renal vasodilation, hyperfiltration, and

reduced myogenic reactivity of small arteries. Circ Res 2003;93:1249–57.

[28] Smith MC, Murdoch AP, Danielson LA, et al. Relaxin has a role in establishing a renal response in pregnancy. Fertil Steril 2006;86:253–5.

[29] Smith MC, Danielson LA, Conrad KP, et al. Influence of recombinant human relaxin on renal hemodynamics in healthy volunteers. J Am Soc Nephrol 2006;17(11):3192–7.

[30] Erikson MS, Unemori EN. Relaxin clinical trials in systemic sclerosis. In: Tregear GW, Ivell R, Bathgate RA, et al, editors. Relaxin. Kluwer Academic Publishers; 2000. p. 373–81.

[31] Dunlop W, Davison JM. The effect of normal pregnancy upon the renal handling of uric acid. Br J Obstet Gynaecol 1977;84:13–21.

[32] Semple PF, Carswell W, Boyle JA. Serial studies of the renal clearance of urate and inulin during pregnancy and after the puerperium in normal women. Clin Sci Mol Med 1974;47:559–65.

[33] Schackis RC. Hyperuricaemia and preeclampsia: is there a pathogenic link? Med Hypotheses 2004;63: 239–44.

[34] Lam C, Lim KH, Kang DH, et al. Uric acid and preeclampsia. Semin Nephrol 2005;25:56–60.

[35] Moran P, Lindheimer MD, Davison JM. The renal response to preeclampsia. Semin Nephrol 2004;24: 588–95.

[36] Thangaratinam S, Ismail KM, Sharp S, et al. Tests in Prediction of Pre-eclampsia Severity Review Group. Accuracy of serum uric acid in predicting complications of pre-eclampsia: a systematic review. BJOG 2006;113:369–78.

[37] Roberts JM, Bodnar LM, Lain KY, et al. Uric acid is as important as proteinuria in identifying fetal risk in women with gestational hypertension. Hypertension 2005;46:1263–9 [see comment].

[38] Taylor AA, Davison JM. Albumin excretion in normal pregnancy. Am J Obstet Gynecol 1997;177: 1559–60 [see comment].

[39] Lopez-Espinoza I, Dhar H, Humphreys S, et al. Urinary albumin excretion in pregnancy. Br J Obstet Gynaecol 1986;93:176–81.

[40] Higby K, Suiter CR, Phelps JY, et al. Normal values of urinary albumin and total protein excretion during pregnancy. Am J Obstet Gynecol 1994;171:984–9.

[41] Bernard A, Thielemans N, Lauwerys R, et al. Selective increase in the urinary excretion of protein 1 (Clara cell protein) and other low molecular weight proteins during normal pregnancy. Scand J Clin Lab Invest 1992;52:871–8.

[42] Hibbard JU, Shroff SG, Lang RM. Cardiovascular changes in preeclampsia. Semin Nephrol 2004;24: 580–7.

[43] Chesney R. Specific renal tubular disorders. In: Goldman L, Ausiello D, editors. Cecil textbook of medicine. Philadelphia: Saunders-Elsevier; 2004. p. 745.

[44] Brenner A. Brenner and Rector's The kidney. Philadelphia: Saunders-Elsevier; 2004.

[45] Davison JM, Hytten FE. The effect of pregnancy on the renal handling of glucose. Br J Obstet Gynaecol 1975;82:374–81.

[46] Bishop JH, Green R. Glucose handling by distal portions of the nephron during pregnancy in the rat. J Physiol 1983;336:131–42.

ELSEVIER
SAUNDERS

Urol Clin N Am 34 (2007) 7–12

UROLOGIC
CLINICS
of North America

Anatomic and Functional Changes of the Lower Urinary Tract During Pregnancy

Mary P. FitzGerald, MD[a],*, Scott Graziano, MD[b]

[a]Division of Female Pelvic Medicine and Reconstructive Surgery, Departments of Urology
and Obstetrics/Gynecology, Loyola University Medical Center, 2160 South First Avenue, Bldg 1003,
Room 1004, Maywood, IL, 60153, USA
[b]Department of Obstetrics/Gynecology, Loyola University Medical Center, 2160 South First Avenue,
Bldg 1003, Room 1004, Maywood, IL, 60153, USA

Bladder anatomy and support in pregnancy

The changes in renal function and upper urinary tract anatomy that occur during pregnancy have been well documented and are presented in another article of this issue. Briefly, there is increased glomerular filtration, increased urinary output, and dilation of the upper tracts. In contrast, relatively little has been published concerning expected alterations in bladder anatomy during pregnancy. Cystoscopically, an indentation of the bladder dome by the enlarged uterus is visible during pregnancy, and the ureteric orifices are visualized in a higher position than in the nonpregnant state [1]. During fluoroscopy, dramatic alterations in the bladder profile can be seen (Fig. 1) [2].

Vaginal delivery is accepted as a major factor predisposing women to prolapse of the pelvic organs [3], including loss of support for the anterior vaginal wall and bladder. Also, there is reasonable evidence to support the belief that it is not vaginal delivery alone, but also pregnancy per se that is associated with increased mobility and descent of the bladder and other pelvic organs. Dietz and colleagues [4] found that at term, the bladder neck descends with Valsalva approximately 5 mm more in pregnant women than in nonpregnant controls, and O'Boyle and coworkers [5,6] found that almost half of primiparous women have pelvic organ prolapse stage 2

(the leading edge of the vaginal walls or cervix come to at least within 1cm of the hymen).

Descent of the anterior vaginal wall and bladder to the level of the hymen by the third trimester of pregnancy can be treated as a normal occurrence in pregnancy, is usually asymptomatic, and usually resolves after delivery. As such, the presence of anterior vaginal wall descent or "cystocele" in this setting does not merit investigation or treatment.

Urinary retention in pregnancy

Although urinary retention is an uncommon urologic emergency, occurring in about 1 in 3000 to 1 in 8000 pregnancies [7,8], instances of urinary retention are seen once or twice per year in the emergency department of any busy hospital. Classically, urinary retention occurs at 12 to 14 weeks of gestation in a retroverted uterus (Fig. 2) [9], with predisposing factors thought to include the presence of uterine fibroids [10], uterine anomalies, and a contracted pelvis [11]. Similar retention episodes also can be seen in women with retroverted, nonpregnant, fibroid uteri that become incarcerated beneath the sacral promontory. Several reports of acute retention in pregnancy make special note of the fact that passage of a catheter in these patients is not difficult, suggesting that compression of the urethra per se is not the cause of retention; Francis [2] proposed that because the bladder base is elevated or stretched, there was failure of relaxation of the urethra during attempts to void (with persistence of the posterior

---

* Corresponding author.
E-mail address: Mfitzg8@lumc.edu (M.P. FitzGerald).

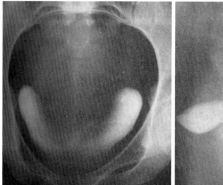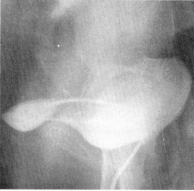

Fig. 1. (*left*) Fluoroscopic image of the bladder in a woman at 14 weeks' gestation, with distortion of the bladder dome by the gravid uterus. There is lateral expansion of the bladder. (*right*) Fluoroscopic image of the bladder in a woman at term. The gravid uterus distorts the bladder, giving it an hourglass shape. (*From* Francis WJA. Disturbances of bladder function in relation to pregnancy. J Obstet Gynaecol Br Empire 1960;67:353–66; with permission.)

urethrovesical angle, at that time considered to be an important finding even in the nonpregnant state). Urodynamic tests done in this setting apparently all have shown an inability to void, lack of urethral relaxation, and no detrusor contraction and have not been clinically useful.

Several lines of evidence suggest but do not prove that progesterone may promote relaxation of bladder smooth muscle and, in extreme cases, detrusor inactivity and retention. Increased bladder capacity and urinary retention was noted when rats received high doses of progesterone [12]. There also have been case reports of patients who had urinary retention after the use of assisted reproductive technology, and who had extremely high progesterone levels but who were not pregnant and who did not have pelvic masses [13]. These patients underwent urodynamic testing and showed no urethral relaxation or detrusor contraction during attempts to void.

Rare instances of uterine incarceration during the third trimester of pregnancy have been reported [14] and are thought to be especially associated with uterine malformations (eg, bicornuate uterus) or abnormal placentation (eg, placenta accreta) in a retroverted uterus. Clinical findings include a failure of fundal height to increase with gestation, and the presence of a fixed mass (the fetus) in the cul-de-sac. Delivery is typically by cesarean section.

Treatment of acute urinary retention during pregnancy is by bladder drainage and bimanual

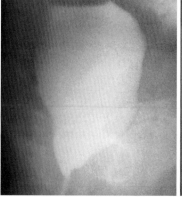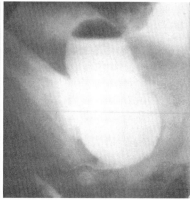

Fig. 2. (*left*) Lateral fluoroscopic image of the bladder in a woman with urinary retention at 14 weeks' gestation with a retroverted uterus, attempting to void. (*right*) Same patient, voiding after placement of a level pessary to antevert the uterus. (*From* Francis WJA. Disturbances of bladder function in relation to pregnancy. J Obstet Gynaecol Br Empire 1960;67:353–66; with permission.)

manipulation of the uterus into an anteverted position with the patient in lithotomy or knee-chest position (occasionally requiring anesthesia for manipulation and, rarely, requiring laparotomy to achieve anteversion). When elevated out of the sacral hollow, the uterus remains in an anteverted position without further intervention in many cases. In other patients, however, the uterus tends to return to the retroverted, presacral position and requires the use of intermittent or continuous catheterization for 1 to 2 weeks until the uterus is large enough that it cannot become incarcerated in the sacral hollow. The temporary use of a Smith-Hodge lever pessary as needed to maintain anteversion of the uterus also is recommended.

Lower urinary tract symptoms

From early pregnancy onward, there is an increase in renal glomerular filtration rate and urine output, and with the fatigue of pregnancy more time is spent in bed at night so that urinary frequency and nocturia can be increased dating from the first weeks of pregnancy. It is tempting also to attribute the observed increase in urinary frequency to the currently fashionable exhortations in lay publications that one should drink "at least 8 to 10 glasses of water daily" while pregnant (there are currently no formal medical guidelines or recommendations with regard to fluid intake during pregnancy), but the fact that 50-year old observations exist about increased urinary frequency during pregnancy suggests that fashionable increases in fluid intake are not the main factor promoting increased urinary frequency during pregnancy.

In 1960, Francis [2] reported that pregnant women had a fluid intake that was an average of 400 to 500 mL greater than nonpregnant controls (presumably in response to homeostatic mechanisms affected by increased fluid output), which may account for some of the increased urinary frequency. Common sense also suggests that simple crowding of the pelvis by the enlarged uterus or descent of the presenting part with fetal engagement during late pregnancy would lead to a decrease in bladder capacity and an increase in urinary frequency. As detailed subsequently, however, cystometric bladder capacity probably does not decrease during pregnancy in most women. Although many observational studies conducted over the last 150 years confirm that urinary symptoms are prevalent in pregnancy, the factors promoting alterations in urinary habits are not fully understood.

Increased urinary frequency is so common in pregnancy that it may reasonably be considered to be a "normal" part of the pregnancy experience. In his 1960 study of 400 pregnant women, Francis [2] found that frequency (defined by seven or more diurnal voids or one or more nocturnal voids) was present at some stage of pregnancy in 81% of women, with most women reporting increased frequency during day and night. He also noted that the first trimester was the usual time for frequency to begin, and that once present, frequency usually became gradually worse as the pregnancy progressed.

Stanton and colleagues [15] carefully studied the development and resolution of urinary symptoms during pregnancy in 83 nulliparae and 98 multiparae. As detailed in Table 1, symptoms of frequency, nocturia, and incontinence all increased throughout pregnancy in primigravidae and multigravidae and generally were found to return toward prepregnancy levels after delivery apart from a persistent elevation in the prevalence of stress and urge incontinence in primigravidae.

Aslan and associates [16] compared lower urinary tract symptoms of 256 pregnant women with 230 nonpregnant controls of similar age, using a validated 7-item questionnaire that asked about voiding, urinary frequency, urgency, and nocturia. Urinary frequency and nocturia showed the greatest increase with each trimester of pregnancy: By the third trimester, mean nocturnal frequency was 2.3 voids per night, with only 14% of pregnant women indicating they did not have any nocturia and 20% indicating they voided three or more times nightly. By the third trimester, 48% of pregnant women had a symptom score that indicated "moderate" or "severe" urinary symptoms compared with 27% of nonpregnant controls of similar age. In contrast, obstructive symptoms were relatively uncommon and varied little as pregnancy progressed.

A notable and consistent finding is that symptoms begin early in pregnancy and persist throughout pregnancy; Cutner and coworkers [17] assessed urinary symptoms in 47 women terminating pregnancy in the first trimester and reported that 19 (40%) complained of urinary frequency, and 29 (62%) had urgency. By the second half of pregnancy [18], 46% of patients had frequency, 57% had nocturia, and 71% had urgency, prevalences that likely differ from those of Stanton's because of differing definitions, study

Table 1
Prevalence (%) of frequency, nocturia, and incontinence during pregnancy in 181 pregnant women (83 primigravid, 98 multigravid)*

	Frequency		Nocturia		Stress incontinence		Urge incontinence	
	Primigravid	Multigravid	Primigravid	Multigravid	Primigravid	Multigravid	Primigravid	Multigravid
Before pregnancy	25	8	4	3	0	10	4	3
At time of first prenatal visit	49	41	19	24	6	26	2	5
At 32 weeks' gestation	67	56	43	37	30	41	10	16
At 40 weeks' gestation	95	76	72	56	34	38	5	20
Postnatal	22	13	6	5	6	11	9	7

* Frequency is defined as voiding >7 times per day, nocturia is defined as voiding ≥2 times at night. The prevalence of all symptoms increases during pregnancy, and except for incontinence in primigravidae, essentially returns to prepregnancy levels in the postpartum period.
  Data from Stanton SL; Kerr-Wilson R, Harris VG. The incidence of urological symptoms in normal pregnancy. Br J Obstet Gynaecol 1980;87:897–900.

methods, and patient population. Similarly Van Brummen and colleagues [19] reported that among 515 nulliparous pregnant women, 74% experienced urinary frequency and 63% experienced urgency by 12 weeks' gestation, increasing to a prevalence of 81% and 68% by 36 weeks.

Lower urinary tract symptoms of frequency, urgency, and nocturia are the norm during pregnancy. There is no recommendation for their treatment, apart from ascertainment that fluid intake is not inappropriately high, and most women are willing to put up with their symptoms when they are reassured that they are likely to resolve soon after delivery.

Urinary incontinence

Urinary incontinence is common in pregnant women and has an impact on quality of life. As detailed in Table 1, urge and stress incontinence occur, with most studies finding that stress incontinence is more common than urge incontinence, although mixed symptoms are frequent [20]. Similar to the onset of other lower urinary tract symptoms, incontinence can begin early and increases significantly in prevalence during pregnancy. In their study of 515 primigravid women, Van Brummen and colleagues [19] found that 6% had symptoms of urge incontinence by 12 weeks, increasing to almost 20% at 36 weeks. In another article, the same authors [16] reported results that are of special interest because they separated the symptoms and life impact that arose from symptoms of

incontinence from other lower urinary tract symptoms that occur during pregnancy. Studying 344 nulliparous women and defining overactive bladder according to women's responses to the Urogenital Distress Inventory, Van Brummen and colleagues [16] found that symptoms of urgency, frequency, and urge incontinence ("wet overactive bladder") increased from a prevalence of 3% at 12 weeks to 15% at 36 weeks of gestation and were associated with an adverse impact on quality of life. Although symptoms of urgency and frequency without leakage ("dry overactive bladder") were more common, being present in 47% of women at 12 weeks and 45% at 36 weeks, they were associated with no significant impact on quality of life.

Dolan and associates [21] also studied the impact of incontinence on quality of life: 36% of 492 primigravidae had incontinence at 36 weeks' gestation, which adversely affected quality of life "moderately" or "a lot" in 13% of women. In Aslan's study [16] alluded to earlier, almost half of pregnant women were "mostly dissatisfied" with their urinary symptoms, and one in five women reported their quality of life as "terrible" if symptoms were to continue.

For treatment of urinary incontinence during pregnancy, most clinicians advise pelvic floor rehabilitation, which can be undertaken through home exercise programs or under formal supervision by a physical therapist. Many women have symptoms that are mild and are simply reassured that incontinence resolves after delivery in most women. There is some evidence that pelvic floor strengthening during pregnancy can prevent incontinence during pregnancy and in the early postpartum period. Morkved and colleagues [22] randomly assigned 301 women in their first pregnancy to attend a 12-week course of physical therapy or to have usual care (no extra pelvic floor strengthening). Significantly fewer women in the pelvic floor training group reported urinary incontinence at 36 weeks' gestation (32% with incontinence in the training group, 48% in the control group) and 3 months postpartum (20% in the training group, 32% in the control group).

The urinary incontinence symptoms of pregnancy persist in the postpartum period in a significant minority of women. In Burgio and colleagues'[23] cohort of 523 women followed for 12 months after delivery, incontinence during pregnancy doubled the odds of urinary incontinence 1 year later. Similarly, when Viktrup [24] studied 278 primiparae, he found that the presence of stress incontinence during the first pregnancy was a strong predictor of stress incontinence symptoms 5 years later. Although it remains to be proven by formal study, it is possible that the occurrence of urinary incontinence during pregnancy should prompt early intervention to prevent the persistence of symptoms.

Urodynamic studies during pregnancy

Because the urinary symptoms of pregnancy begin early and are not easily explained by current models, several investigators have undertaken urodynamic testing to examine bladder physiology during pregnancy in detail. Results of urodynamic studies during pregnancy are contradictory.

Reports of increased bladder compliance and "atony" during pregnancy appeared in 1939, when Muellner [25] reported his findings in 50 (presumably, asymptomatic) pregnant women studied with single-channel cystometry as their bladders were filled with increments of 50 mL of warm boric acid solution. He found that "starting at the third month of pregnancy, the bladder capacity slowly increases, reaching its largest limits, up to 1300cc in the eighth month … in the third trimester (the bladder) shows definite evidence of atony…. At this time the bladder sensations are not as clear-cut as in the non-pregnant control." Muellner [25] reported that although elevated postvoid residual urine volumes were common in the immediate postpartum period, bladder

function had returned to normal by 6 to 8 weeks postpartum.

In contrast, using multichannel urodynamic testing in 14 continent primigravid women, Iosif and coworkers [26] found that bladder pressure at maximum capacity increased from an average of 9 cm H_2O during the second trimester to 20 cm H_2O at the end of pregnancy ($P<.001$) and returned to normal after delivery. The increase in bladder pressure was attributed to the presence of the enlarged uterus. Similar findings have been reported in other studies [27,28], but in contrast, Francis [2] found no difference in the bladder capacity of pregnant women and found that women with the greatest bladder capacities complained of the greatest urinary frequency.

Iosif's study [26] found that in continent pregnant women, functional urethral length, maximal urethral pressure, and closure pressure increased (by an average of 12 cm H_2O) during pregnancy and returned to normal during the first week after vaginal delivery. Iosif and colleagues [27] and Van Geelen and associates[28] reported that pregnant women with stress incontinence had lower functional urethral lengths and closure pressures than the continent controls, with Iosif's group finding that stress incontinent women did not show the same increase in functional urethral length as the women who were continent.

Nel and coworkers [29] assessed 40 patients with multichannel urodynamic testing during and after pregnancy and found urodynamic stress incontinence in 12% during pregnancy and in none after pregnancy. Detrusor instability was found in 23% during pregnancy and in 15% after pregnancy, with all patients who had detrusor instability postpartum showing detrusor instability during pregnancy. No information about prepregnancy symptoms was given. Finally, Cutner and associates [18] studied 28 women with median gestational age of 28 weeks and found detrusor instability in 10 (36%). They found that symptoms of frequency, urgency, and nocturia were no more prevalent in women with detrusor instability than in women who did not show detrusor instability. During pregnancy, urinary symptoms do not correspond to urodynamic findings, and urodynamic testing is not clinically helpful.

Summary

During pregnancy, lower urinary tract function is altered considerably in many women. Normal function apparently returns for most women soon after delivery. It is unclear whether the presence of urinary incontinence during pregnancy is a marker for future development of other pelvic floor disorders and perhaps should lead to consideration of cesarean delivery or perhaps early postpartum rehabilitation of the pelvic floor to prevent those disorders. This and similar questions await formal study.

References

[1] Hundley JMJ, Siegel IA, Hachtel FW, et al. Some physiological and pathological observations on the urinary tract during pregnancy. Surg Gynecol Obstet 1938;66:360–79.

[2] Francis WJA. Disturbances of bladder function in relation to pregnancy. J Obstet Gynecol Br Empire 1960;67:353–66.

[3] Chiaffarino F, Chatenoud L, Dindelli M, et al. Reproductive factors, family history, occupation and risk of urogenital prolapse. Eur J Obstet Gynaecol Reprod Biol 1999;82:63–7.

[4] Dietz HP, Eldridge A, Grace M, et al. Does pregnancy affect pelvic organ mobility? Aust N Z J Obstet Gynaecol 2004;44:S17–20.

[5] O'Boyle AL, Woodman PJ, O'Boyle JD, et al. Pelvic organ support in nulliparous pregnant and nonpregnant women: a case control study. Am J Obstet Gynecol 2002;187:99–102.

[6] O'Boyle AL, O'Boyle JD, Ricks RE, et al. The natural history of pelvic organ support in pregnancy. Int Urogynecol J 2003;14:46–9.

[7] Keating PJ, Maouris P, Walton SM. Incarceration of a bicornuate retroverted gravid uterus presenting with bilateral ureteric obstruction. Br J Obstet Gynaecol 1992;99:345–7.

[8] Weekes ARL, Atlay RD, Brown VA, et al. The retroverted gravid uterus and its effect on the outcome of pregnancy. BMJ 1976;1:622–4.

[9] Silva PD, Berberich W. Retroverted impacted gravid uterus with acute urinary retention: report of two cases and a review of the literature. J Reprod Med 1986;68:121–3.

[10] Schwartz Z, Dgani R, Katz Z, et al. Urinary retention caused by impaction of leiomyoma in pregnancy. Acta Obstet Gynaecol Scand 1986;65:525–6.

[11] Gibbons JM, Paley WB. The incarcerated gravid uterus. Obstet Gynecol 1969;331:842–5.

[12] Langworthy OR, Brack CB. The effect of pregnancy and the corpus luteum upon vesical muscle. Am J Obstet Gynecol 1939;37:121–5.

[13] Chen Y-J, Chang S-P, Yuan C-C, et al. Acute urinary retention after use of assisted reproductive technology: a report of 2 cases. J Reprod Med 2003;48:560–2.

[14] Van Winter JT, Ogburn PL, Ney JA, et al. Uterine incarceration during the third trimester: a rare complication of pregnancy. Mayo Clin Proc 1991;66:608–13.

[15] Stanton SL, Kerr-Wilson R, Harris VG. The incidence of urological symptoms in normal pregnancy. Br J Obstet Gynaecol 1980;87:897–900.

[16] Aslan D, Aslan G, Yamazhan M, et al. Voiding symptoms in pregnancy: an assessment with International Prostate Symptom Score. Gynecol Obstet Invest 2003;55:46–9.

[17] Cutner A, Cardozo LD, Benness CJ. Assessment of urinary symptoms in early pregnancy. Br J Obstet Gynaecol 1991;98:1283–6.

[18] Cutner A, Cardozo LD, Benness CJ. Assessment of urinary symptoms in the second half of pregnancy. Int Urogynecol J 1992;3:30–2.

[19] Van Brummen HJ, Bruinse HW, Van der Bom JG, et al. How do the prevalences of urogenital symptoms change during pregnancy? Neurourol Urodynam 2006;25:135–9.

[20] Raza-Khan F, Graziano S, Kenton K, et al. Peripartum urinary incontinence in a racially diverse obstetrical population. Int Urogyn J 2006;17:525–30.

[21] Dolan LM, Walsh D, Hamilton S, et al. A study of quality of life in primigravidae with urinary incontinence. Int Urogynecol J 2004;15:160–4.

[22] Morkved S, Bo K, Schei B, et al. Pelvic floor muscle training during pregnancy to prevent urinary incontinence: a single-blind randomized controlled trial. Obstet Gynecol 2003;101:313–9.

[23] Burgio KL, Zyczynski H, Locher JL, et al. Urinary incontinence in the 12-month postpartum period. Obstet Gynecol 2003;6:1291–8.

[24] Viktrup L. The risk of lower urinary tract symptoms five years after the first delivery. Neurourol Urodynam 2002;21:2–29.

[25] Muellner SR. Physiological bladder changes during pregnancy and the puerperium. J Urol 1939;41:691–5.

[26] Iosif S, Ingemarsson I, Ulmsten U. Urodynamic studies in normal pregnancy and in puerperium. Am J Obstet Gynecol 1980;137:696–700.

[27] Iosif S, Ulmsten U. Comparative urodynamic studies of continent and stress incontinent women in pregnancy and in the puerperium. Am J Obstet Gynecol 1981;140:645–50.

[28] Van Geelen JM, Lemmens WAJG, Eskes TKAB, et al. The urethral pressure profile in pregnancy and after delivery in healthy nulliparous women. Am J Obstet Gynecol 1982;144:636–49.

[29] Nel JT, Diedericks A, Joubert G, et al. A prospective clinical and urodynamic study of bladder function during and after pregnancy. Int Urogynecol J 2001;12:21–6.

ELSEVIER
SAUNDERS

Urol Clin N Am 34 (2007) 13–21

UROLOGIC
CLINICS
of North America

Postpartum Genitourinary Changes

Rebecca G. Rogers, MD[a],*, Larry L. Leeman, MD[a,b]

[a]Department of Obstetrics and Gynecology, University of New Mexico Health Sciences Center,
1 University of New Mexico, MSC10 5580, Albuquerque, NM 87131-0001, USA
[b]Department of Family and Community Medicine, University of New Mexico Health Sciences Center,
1 University of New Mexico, MSC10 5580, Albuquerque, NM 87131-0001, USA

Pregnancy and childbirth can affect the lower genitourinary tract through anatomic changes, denervation injury, or traumatic injury. Effects of childbirth are often global, including changes in urinary and anal continence and pelvic floor support. Up to one third of premenopausal women and almost one half of postmenopausal women experience some type of pelvic floor disorder in their lifetime, including urinary or anal incontinence or pelvic organ prolapse [1]. Childbirth or pregnancy have been implicated as antecedents for all three disorders. Causation is difficult to prove because symptoms often occur remote from delivery. It is unclear from current literature whether changes are secondary to the method of childbirth or to the pregnancy itself. This controversy fuels the debate about whether or not women should be offered the choice of elective cesarean delivery to avoid the development of subsequent pelvic floor dysfunction. In this article, we aim to describe genitourinary postpartum pelvic floor changes, and review the literature regarding the impact of pregnancy or childbirth on these changes.

Genital tract trauma

During vaginal birth, most women experience pelvic floor trauma that requires suturing [2]. Episiotomy and operative vaginal delivery increase the incidence of severe pelvic floor trauma and are proven risk factors for subsequent pelvic floor dysfunction, yet they were performed in 29%

and 9% of vaginal births, respectively, in 2001 [3,4]. Genital tract lacerations are graded on a scale of one to four. First-degree lacerations involve only the vaginal mucosa or perineal skin. Second-degree lacerations involve the muscles of the perineal body without transgressing the anal sphincter complex. Third-degree lacerations include any laceration of the external anal sphincter, and fourth-degree lacerations include laceration of the both the internal and external anal sphincter, and the rectal mucosa (Table 1). Aside from the immediate pain and discomfort of perineal lacerations, tears of the anal sphincter complex affect long-term anal continence, with up to 40% of women complaining of anal incontinence following anal sphincter laceration [5]. Sphincter laceration is also associated with a 270% increase in sexual pain postpartum, when compared with women who deliver without perineal laceration [6]. It is better to tear than to be cut; women who deliver with spontaneous lacerations report less pain with intercourse than women who undergo episiotomy. The impact of less severe first- and second-degree laceration on pelvic floor function is unknown.

Denervation injury

The pudendal nerve travels along the posterior wall of the pelvis and ultimately exits the pelvis to innervate the external genitalia. Because of its length and position, it is vulnerable to both compression and stretch injury, particularly during vaginal birth, when the fetal head is compressed against the pelvic floor. Denervation injury has been implicated in postpartum urinary

* Corresponding author.
E-mail address: rrogers@salud.unm.edu (R.G. Rogers).

Table 1
Perineal lacerations

Degree of laceration	Structures Involved
First	Vaginal mucosa, perineal skin
Second	*All above and* muscles of perineum
Third	*All above and* external anal sphincter
Fourth	*All above and* rectal mucosa

and fecal incontinence [7,8]. Assessment of pudendal nerve terminal motor latencies (PNTML) before and after childbirth demonstrates alterations in women after vaginal birth or cesarean delivery after labor. These changes do not appear during pregnancy [9], and often resolve by 6 months after birth [10]. Women assessed 48 hours postpartum have significantly greater prolongation in PNTML when they have had a forceps-assisted vaginal delivery, compared with spontaneous vaginal birth [11].

Pelvic floor muscle injury

Pelvic floor damage from childbirth can be measured objectively by the use of MRI of the levator ani complex. Nulliparous women do not have defects in levator ani musculature as evaluated by MRI. Up to 20% of primiparous women develop defects in the levator ani after vaginal birth [12]. The defects occur most commonly in the pubovisceral portion of the levator ani. The levator ani injuries have been shown to be associated with stress urinary incontinence, but it remains unclear if the defect is responsible for stress incontinence or is simply a marker of global pelvic floor injury. Three-dimensional translabial ultrasound has also been used to demonstrate postpartum levator injury [13].

Urinary incontinence

Stress or urge incontinence before pregnancy or childbirth is rare, occurring in less than 1% of women [14]. Stress urinary incontinence during pregnancy is common, and affects up to 32% of primiparous women [15,16]. The causes of stress incontinence during pregnancy are thought to include maternal weight gain and increased mechanical pressure on the bladder from the enlarging uterus, and increased urine production from increased glomerular filtration rates. Although many women with stress incontinence during pregnancy report resolution of symptoms

postpartum, the presence of incontinence during pregnancy may be predictive of postpartum incontinence [17,18]. Postpartum incontinence in the short term may be predictive of longer-term problems. Women with persistent stress urinary incontinence at 3 months postpartum have a 92% risk of having stress urinary incontinence at 5 years [19]. Cross-sectional [20] and cohort studies [21,22] demonstrate a higher prevalence of stress incontinence in women who have had vaginal deliveries, compared with women only having cesarean deliveries. These differences are significant only in younger women; in older women, the stress incontinence risk factors of age and obesity outweigh the effect of childbirth and method of delivery [23]. A study of urinary incontinence in a cohort of nulliparous nuns with an average age of 68 years demonstrated prevalence rates similar to the general population, suggesting that obstetric history has minimal impact in older women [24]. Women having cesarean delivery after labor appear to have a similar incidence of stress incontinence, compared with women after vaginal birth, suggesting that the labor process, rather than vaginal birth itself, may be implicated in pelvic floor damage [25].

A single randomized controlled trial of vaginal versus cesarean delivery has examined the impact of mode of delivery on the incidence of urinary incontinence. Women who underwent cesarean delivery reported less urinary incontinence than women who delivered vaginally at 3 months postpartum (relative risk 0.62, 95% CI 0.41–0.93) [26], although the difference did not persist 2 years postpartum [27].

Effects of childbirth on urge urinary incontinence are less well described. Urge incontinence may occur as commonly as stress symptoms after childbirth, affecting approximately 30% of postpartum women [14]. Forceps delivery and episiotomy have been associated with increased reports of urge incontinence, whereas cesarean delivery has been protective [14]. Fetal macrosomia has been associated with the development of both stress and urge symptoms [21].

Not all incontinence is troublesome to patients. Most studies evaluating the incidence and impact of postpartum urinary incontinence compare women with any urinary incontinence with women with no incontinence, and do not include descriptions of the severity of incontinence. This omission underlines the importance of using reliable methods of obtaining information regarding functional outcomes. The use of validated and reliable questionnaires to evaluate both symptom severity and quality of life is essential for future evaluation of postpartum pelvic floor changes.

Obstetric fistula

Damage to the bladder or ureters may occur during the process of childbirth. The classic bladder injury is vesicovaginal fistula caused by obstructed labor leading to necrosis of the anterior vaginal wall. Less commonly, rectovaginal fistulas can occur. (Fig. 1) [28]. Although now rare in the developed world, such injuries remain a common source of lifelong morbidity in developing countries. Improved access to cesarean delivery for labor dystocia is preventive. The World Health Organization has estimated that more than 2 million girls and women around the world have unrepaired fistulas, figures that probably underestimate the extent of the disease because they are based on women who present for care [29]. Without repair, these women face the potential for life-long rejection from their families and community because of their incontinence.

Operative injuries

Injury to the bladder and ureters during cesarean delivery is an uncommon cause of urologic injury. The bladder may be lacerated during cesarean delivery at the time of peritoneal entry, development of the bladder flap, incision of

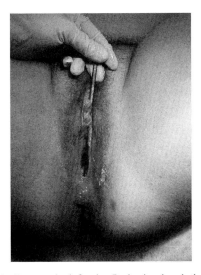

Fig. 1. Rectovaginal fistula. Probe is placed through fistulous tract. (Courtesy of Rebecca G. Rogers, MD, Albuquerque, NM.)

the uterus, or lysis of adhesions. Prior cesarean delivery is associated with increased risk, as is cesarean after onset of labor [30]. Women having a fourth cesarean had a 1.2% risk of bladder injury, compared with 0.13% in a first cesarean delivery [31]. Fortunately, most bladder injuries involve the dome of the bladder, with minimal long-term morbidity if recognized intraoperatively. When bladder laceration is suspected but is not grossly apparent, further evaluation is done by filling the bladder with methylene blue, indigo carmine, or sterile milk, which is readily available on labor and delivery units.

The ureters are rarely transected or occluded during cesarean delivery. The common scenario for ureteral injury is lateral extension of the uterine incision into the broad ligament, with inadvertent ligation of the ureter when hemostatic sutures are placed. Unfortunately, unlike bladder injuries, which are usually detected, these injuries may remain occult. The incidence of ureteral injury is 0.03% in first cesarean deliveries and it remains rare, even in patients who have had multiple prior cesarean deliveries, where the operative field may be obscured by scarring [31].

An Israeli medical center reported urologic consultation in 0.3% of 10,439 cesarean deliveries. Twelve of the twenty-nine consultations were for inadvertent cystotomy and seventeen for possible ureteral injury. Ureteral injuries were confirmed in only two cases: one with inadvertent cystotomy and one with suspected intraoperative ureteral ligation [32].

Postpartum urinary retention

The diagnosis, incidence, and treatment of postpartum urinary retention are controversial, with few studies of this common disorder. A functional definition is the inability to void spontaneously within 6 hours of vaginal delivery, or within 6 hours of the removal of a urinary catheter after cesarean [33]. An alternative definition is based on postvoid residual volume, as assessed by abdominal ultrasound or bladder catheterization. The definition of an abnormal postpartum postvoid residual remains controversial, with the upper threshold varying from 50 to 200 mL. Given these differences in definitions, the incidence of urinary retention in prospective studies has varied from 1.5% to 14% [33]. When a functional definition described above is used, the incidence was 2.1% of vaginal and 3.2% of cesarean deliveries [34]. Risk factors for postpartum urinary retention include nulliparity, prolonged labor, operative vaginal delivery, and possible epidural anesthesia [35]. Postpartum urinary retention may be treated by placement of an indwelling catheter for a period of time (eg, 12–48 hours), or the use of intermittent bladder catheterization every 4 to 6 hours, until the postvoid residual is below 150 mL [33]. One study demonstrated no need for repeat catheterization if the initial postvoid residual was below 700 mL [36].

Careful postpartum care to detect women who are unable to void spontaneously is important. Early detection decreases the proportion of women who require long-term catheterization secondary to extreme bladder overdistention. On the other hand, for women who can void spontaneously, the usefulness of routine screening of postvoid residuals is unclear. One group suggested that routine screening might be beneficial. In their study, 85 women had bladder ultrasound within 6 hours postpartum. Twenty-seven (32%) had postvoid residuals of more than 300 mL. Of these, only 17 would have been suspected, based on signs or symptoms [37]. In contrast, other groups did not find routine ultrasound screening to be effective. In one study of 707 women, 34 (4.9%) had symptomatic urinary retention, and 67 (9.7%) had no symptoms but had residuals of more than 150 mL on postpartum day 1. Of these 67 women, all improved spontaneously with postvoid residuals of less than 150 mL by postpartum day 4 [38]. Four years later, the subjects were recontacted, and voiding symptoms were similar for the women with, versus without, postpartum retention. In the follow-up study, the investigators did not separate the women with symptomatic retention from those with high postvoid residuals found by screening [39]. Another group also doubted the usefulness of routine screening. In their study of 543 women, 4 had frank postpartum retention and 8 had postvoid residuals of more than 150 mL on postpartum day 3. By day 5, all eight had improved spontaneously, with postvoid residuals of less than 150 mL. Ten of the twelve subjects with retention were available for follow-up 4 years later, and none had any voiding difficulty [40]. These three studies all indicate that the incidence of postpartum retention decreases greatly as the time from delivery increased.

Anal incontinence

Anal incontinence, or the loss of flatus, formed, or loose stool that is a social or hygienic problem, can occur secondary to pregnancy or childbirth [41]. The anal sphincter complex includes the internal and external anal sphincters and the rectal mucosa, and lies in close proximity to the puborectalis (Fig. 2). The complex extends for a distance of 3 cm up the anal canal. The striated muscle of the external anal sphincter is responsible for the squeeze tone of the anal canal, but only 10% to 20% of the resting tone. The internal anal sphincter, which is made up of smooth muscle, provides 80% to 90% of the resting tone of the anus [42]. Because of its proximity to the perineal body, the anal sphincter complex is vulnerable to damage at childbirth. Damage can occur after laceration of the anal sphincters, and from nerve or muscle damage during vaginal birth. Vaginal birth leads to overt anal sphincter laceration in up to 6% of women [43–46]. Despite repair, 20% to 50% of these women complain of involuntary loss of flatus or stool [47–50].

Up to 30% of sphincter injuries are detectable only with ultrasonography of the anal sphincter complex and are not associated with overt perineal laceration [51]. These hidden lacerations may account for the 13% of women who report symptoms of anal incontinence without a history of sphincter laceration. Because of occult injury, the incidence of anal sphincter damage at the time of vaginal delivery is higher than the number of observed injuries would suggest [48]. Identification of these occult sphincter lacerations by postpartum ultrasound may be beneficial to parturients. In a recent randomized trial, severe anal incontinence 1 year after delivery was reduced in women who underwent repair of occult laceration identified by ultrasound [52].

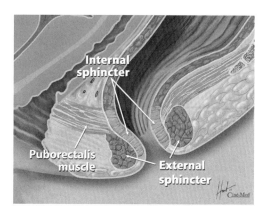

Fig. 2. Obstetric anal sphincter anatomy. (Courtesy of Cine-Med, Inc., Woodbury, CT; with permission. © Cine-Med, Inc.)

Episiotomy and operative vaginal delivery are known risk factors in the development of anal incontinence symptoms [45]. A meta-analysis of six randomized trials compared restrictive to liberal use of episiotomy in 4850 women, and concluded that liberal use of episiotomies conferred no benefit [53]. Operative vaginal delivery was reviewed similarly in 2582 women and it was found that vacuum delivery was associated with a much lower risk of anal sphincter laceration than delivery with forceps (relative risk 0.41, 95% CIs 0.33 to 0.50) [54]. The incidence of anal incontinence following sphincter laceration increases over time. For example, in a cohort of 72 women who had anal sphincter laceration, 4% had stool incontinence at 3 months after delivery, and this increased to 17% 2 to 4 years later [55]. Prevention of anal sphincter laceration and subsequent development of anal incontinence partly lies in decreasing the use of episiotomy and forceps delivery at the time of delivery.

Surprisingly, cesarean delivery does not necessarily prevent postpartum anal incontinence symptoms. In the randomized Term Breech trial, the incidence of fecal incontinence at 2-year follow-up was approximately 2% for women in both the vaginal birth and cesarean birth groups, and the incidence of flatal incontinence was approximately 10% in both groups [27]. In a cohort study that compared women after elective cesarean delivery, planned cesarean delivery, or noninstrumental vaginal delivery, the incidences of fecal incontinence were similar for all three groups [56]. These findings suggest that some anal incontinence symptoms may be caused by pregnancy itself; in fact, 8% to 42% of women have mild anal incontinence symptoms before their first vaginal delivery [50,57]. However, the pathophysiology of how pregnancy per se would affect anal continence is undefined.

The most common cause of anal incontinence in young women is anal sphincter injury at childbirth. With advancing age, like urinary incontinence, the affects of childbirth may be superseded by other risk factors, such as aging [58].

Pelvic organ prolapse

Pelvic organ prolapse is the herniation of the pelvic organs to or through the vaginal opening (Fig. 3). Approximately 300,000 pelvic organ prolapse operations are performed yearly in the United States, and these surgeries outnumber surgery for stress incontinence by a 2:1 ratio. One in

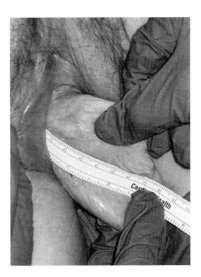

Fig. 3. Pelvic organ prolapse. The vagina is completely turned inside out. (Courtesy of Rebecca G. Rogers, MD, Albuquerque, NM.)

nine women will have surgery for pelvic floor disorders by age 80, and 30% will require reoperation [59–61]. Symptoms of pelvic organ prolapse include bulge symptoms, urinary or bowel symptoms, sexual symptoms, and pain [62].

Risk factors for development of pelvic organ prolapse are multifactorial, and include pregnancy, vaginal birth, aging, increased intra-abdominal pressure, menopause, hypoestrogenism, trauma, genetic factors, race, musculoskeletal diseases, chronic diseases, smoking, and prior surgery [63]. Vaginal delivery is the risk factor cited most commonly for the development of pelvic organ prolapse, and is supported by observations from epidemiologic studies. In the Oxford family planning study, women with two deliveries were 8.4 times more likely to have surgery for prolapse, compared with women with no deliveries [64]. More recently, a survey of 4458 women found that vaginal parity compared with cesarean delivery was associated with an increased odds ratio for prolapse of 1.82 (95% CI 1.04–3.19) [65].

Prolapse can occur during pregnancy; up to 46% of nulliparous women have been shown to have some prolapse in the late third trimester [66]. Other studies have demonstrated that bladder and urethral mobility increase in pregnancy. These changes are greatest in the third trimester [67].

Sexual function

Most women resume sexual activity by 8 weeks postpartum, and nearly all have some sexual complaints [68]. Only 14% of women and 12% of men report no sexual problems whatsoever postpartum [69]. Six months postpartum, 35% of primiparous women complain of decreased sexual sensation and 24% of decreased sexual satisfaction, compared with function before childbirth. In the same retrospective cohort, 22% also complained of dyspareunia [6]. Intercourse-related problems can persist 12 to 18 months following delivery [70], and are more common in women who underwent operative vaginal delivery [71]. Women who have episiotomies or spontaneous perineal lacerations complain of increased perineal pain [72], decreased sexual satisfaction postpartum, and delayed return of sexual activity, compared with women who give birth with an intact perineum [71,73]. Women with severe perineal lacerations of the anal sphincter are more likely to report dyspareunia than women with an intact perineum [6].

It is unclear whether or not cesarean delivery is protective of postpartum sexual complaints. Because cesarean delivery avoids genital tract trauma, it has often been assumed to protect sexual function postpartum [74]. Some investigators have found that increased reports of pain are limited to the immediate postpartum timeframe, with differences between cesarean and vaginal delivery groups resolving by 6 months postpartum [74]. Nearly all studies that have examined the effect of mode of delivery on postpartum sexual complaints conclude that sexual dysfunction is highest in women undergoing operative vaginal delivery with forceps or vacuum [75].

Elective primary cesarean delivery

Does elective cesarean delivery prevent the development of pelvic floor disorders? The National Institute of Health held a consensus conference titled "Cesarean Delivery on Maternal Request" in March 2006 to address this question [76]. Although some pelvic floor disorders seem to be reduced in women who undergo elective cesarean delivery, the quality of the evidence supporting this was assessed as weak. Of particular concern in the consensus statement was how long differences between vaginal and cesarean delivery persisted, and the potential impact of multiple cesarean deliveries on the development of pelvic floor disorders. For example, a comparison of women who underwent three cesarean deliveries with women after three vaginal births showed comparable rates of stress urinary incontinence, perhaps because of the cumulative effect of pregnancy itself or denervation injury during cesarean delivery [77].

When comparing elective cesarean to vaginal delivery, it is important to appreciate that all vaginal deliveries may not be equivalent in their impact on the pelvic floor. A style of actively coached pushing was associated with increased urge incontinence at 3 months, when compared with women who were not actively coached [78]. Much can be done to prevent pelvic floor disorders by limiting the use of episiotomy and operative delivery using forceps, known risk factors for pelvic floor dysfunction. One can learn from past mistakes. Episiotomy was adopted in the 1920s to protect the pelvic floor, without clear evidence to support its use [79]. Years later, one third of women still undergo episiotomy, despite lack of evidence of benefit, and risk of significant harm [80]. What is needed before making broad public health changes in delivery method is data comparing the effects of pregnancy alone, cesarean delivery (labored and unlabored), and vaginal birth. Perhaps then, physicians will have better information to help advise patients about the postpartum genitourinary tract changes they might expect.

References

[1] Brown JS, Posner SF, Stewart AL. Urge incontinence: new health-related quality of life measures. J Am Geriatr Soc 1999;47(8):980–8.
[2] Albers L, Garcia J, Renfrew M, et al. Distribution of genital tract trauma in childbirth and related postnatal pain. Birth 1999;26:11–5.
[3] Kozak LJ, Owings MF, Hall MJ. National hospital discharge survey: 2001 annual summary with detailed diagnosis and procedure data. Vital Health Stat 13 2004 Jun;(156):1–198.
[4] Martin JA, Hamilton BE, Sutton PD, et al. Births: final data for 2002. Natl Vital Stat Rep 2003;52(10).
[5] Garcia V, Rogers RG, Kim SS, et al. Primary repair of obstetric anal sphincter laceration: a randomized trial of two surgical techniques. Am J Obstet Gynecol 2005;192(5):1697–701.
[6] Signorello LB, Harlow BL, Chekos AK, et al. Postpartum sexual functioning and its relationship to perineal trauma: a retrospective cohort study of primiparous women. Am J Obstet Gynecol 2001; 184(5):881–90.
[7] Snooks SJ, Setchell M, Swash M, et al. Injury to innervation of pelvic floor sphincter musculature in childbirth. Lancet 1984;2:546–50.
[8] Snooks SJ, Swash M, Mathers SE, et al. Effect of vaginal delivery on the pelvic floor: a 5-year follow-up. Br J Surg 1990;77:1358–60.

[9] Tetzschner T, Sorensen M, Lose G, et al. Pudendal nerve function during pregnancy and after delivery. Int Urogynecol J Pelvic Floor Dysfunct 1997;8(2): 66–8.

[10] Sultan AH, Kamm MA, Hudson CN. Pudendal nerve damage during labour: prospective study before and after childbirth. BJOG 1994;101:22–8.

[11] Snooks SJ, Swash M, Henry MM, et al. Risk factors in childbirth causing damage to the pelvic floor innervation. Int J Colorectal Dis 1986;1:20–4.

[12] DeLancey JOL, Kearney R, Chou Q, et al. The appearance of levator ani muscle abnormalities in magnetic resonance images after vaginal delivery. Obstet Gynecol 2003;101:46–53.

[13] Dietz HP, Lanzarone V. Levator trauma after vaginal delivery. Obstet Gynecol 2005;106:707–12.

[14] Casey BM, Schaffer JI, Bloom SL, et al. Obstetric antecedents for postpartum pelvic floor dysfunction. Am J Obstet Gynecol 2005;192:1655–62.

[15] Viktrup L. The symptom of stress incontinence caused by pregnancy or delivery in primiparas. Obstet Gynecol 1992;79:945–9.

[16] Thorp JM, Norton PA, Wall LL, et al. Urinary incontinence in pregnancy and the puerperium: a prospective study. Am J Obstet Gynecol 1999;181:266–73.

[17] van Brummen HJ, Bruinse HW, van de Pol G, et al. The effect of vaginal and cesarean delivery on lower urinary tract symptoms: what makes the difference. Int Urogynecol J Pelvic Floor Dysfunct 2006; [Epub ahead of print].

[18] Foldspang A, Hvidman A, Mommsen S, et al. Risk of postpartum urinary incontinence associated with pregnancy and mode of delivery. Acta Obstat Gynecol Scand 2004;83:923–7.

[19] Viktrup L, Lose G. The risk of stress incontinence 5 years after first delivery. Am J Obstet Gynecol 2001;185:82–7.

[20] Persson J, Wolner-hanssen P, Rydhstroem H. Obstetric risk factors for stress urinary incontinence: a population-based study. Obstet Gynecol 2000;96:440–5.

[21] Rortveit G, Daltveit AK, Hannestad YS, et al. Norwegian EPINCONT study. Urinary incontinence after vaginal delivery or cesarean section. N Engl J Med 2003;348:900–7.

[22] Burgio KL, Zyczynski H, Locher JL, et al. Urinary incontinence in the 12-month postpartum period. Obstet Gynecol 2003;102:1291–8.

[23] Fritel X, Ringa V, Varnoux N, et al. Mode of delivery and severe stress incontinence: a cross-sectional study among 2625 perimenopausal women. BJOG 2005;112:1–6.

[24] Buchsbaum GM, Chin M, Glantz C, et al. Prevalence of urinary incontinence and associated risk factors in a cohort of nuns. Obstet Gynecol 2002;100:226–9.

[25] Groutz A, Rimon E, Peled S, et al. Cesarean section: does it really prevent the development of postpartum stress urinary incontinence? A prospective study of 363 women one year after their first delivery. Neurourol Urodynam 2004;23:2–6.

[26] Hannah ME, Hannah WJ, Hodnett ED, et al. Term breech trial 3-month follow-up collaborative group. Outcomes at 3 months after planned cesarean vs. planned vaginal delivery for breech presentation at term: The International Randomized Term Breech Trial. JAMA 2002;287:1822–31.

[27] Hannah ME, Whyte H, Hannah WJ, et al. Maternal outcomes at 2 years after planned cesarean section versus planned vaginal birth for breech presentation at term: The International Randomized Term Breech Trial. Am J Obstet Gynecol 2004;191:917–27.

[28] Wall LL, Arrowsmith SD, Briggs ND, et al. The obstetric vesicovaginal fistula in the developing world. Obstet Gynecol Surv 2005;60(7):S3–51.

[29] Murray C, Lopez A. Health dimensions of sex and reproduction. Geneva (Switzerland): WHO; 1998.

[30] Phipps MG, Watabe B, Clemons JL, et al. Risk factors for bladder injury during cesarean delivery. Obstet Gynecol 2005;105:156–60.

[31] Silver RM, Landon MB, Rouse DJ, et al. Maternal morbidity associated with multiple repeat cesarean deliveries. Obstet Gynecol 2006;107:1226–32.

[32] Yossepowitch O, Baniel J, Livne P. Urological injuries during cesarean section: intraoperative diagnosis and management. J Urol 2004;172:196–9.

[33] Yip S, Sahota D, Pang M, et al. Postpartum urinary retention. Acta Obstet Gynecol Scand 2004;83: 881–91.

[34] Kermans G, Wyndaele JJ, Thiery M, et al. Puerperal urinary retention. Acta Urol Belg 1986;54:376–85.

[35] Yip S, Sahota D, Pang M, et al. Postpartum urinary retention. Obstet Gynecol 2005;106:602–6.

[36] Burkhart FL, Porges RF, Gibbs CF. Bladder capacity postpartum and catheterization. Obstet Gynecol 1965;26:176–9.

[37] Van Os AF, Van der Linden PJ. Reliability of an automatic ultrasound system in the post partum period in measuring urinary retention. Acta Obstet Gynecol Scand 2006;85:604–7.

[38] Yip SK, Brieger G, Hin LY, et al. Urinary retention in the post-partum period. The relationship between obstetric factors and the post-partum post-void residual bladder volume. Acta Obstet Gynecol Scand 1997;76:667–72.

[39] Yip S, Sahota D, Chang AMZ, et al. Four-year follow-up of women who were diagnosed to have postpartum urinary retention. Am J Obstet Gynecol 2002;187:648–52.

[40] Andolf E, Iosif CS, Jorgensen C, et al. Insidious urinary retention after vaginal delivery: prevalence and symptoms at follow-up in a population-based study. Gynecol Obstet Unvest 1994;38:51–3.

[41] Norton C, Christianson I, Butler U, et al. Anal incontinence. In: Abrams P, Cardozo L, Khoury S, et al, editors. Incontinence. 2nd edition: International consultation on incontinence, 2001. Paris: Health publications, Ltd; 2002.

[42] Delancey JOL, Toglia MR, Perucchini D. Internal and external anal sphincter anatomy as it relates to

midline obstetric lacerations. Obstet Gynecol 1997; 90:924–7.

[43] Sultan AH, Kamm MA, Hudson CN, et al. Anal sphincter disruption during vaginal delivery. N Engl J Med 1993;329:1905–11.

[44] Handa VL, Danielson BH, Gilbert WM. Obstetric anal sphincter lacerations. Obstet Gynecol 2001;98: 225–30.

[45] Eason E, Labrecque M, Marcoux S, et al. Anal incontinence after childbirth. CMAJ 2002;166:326–30.

[46] Zetterstrom J, Lopez A, Anzen B, et al. Anal sphincter tears at vaginal delivery: risk factors and clinical outcome of primary repair. Obstet Gynecol 1999;94:21–8.

[47] Fitzpatrick M, Behan M, O'Connell PR, et al. A randomized clinical trial comparing primary overlap with approximation repair of third-degree obstetric tears. Am J Obstet Gynecol 2000;183:1220–4.

[48] Varma A, Gunn J, Gardiner A, et al. Obstetrical anal sphincter injury: prospective evaluation and incidence. Dis Colon Rectum 1999;42:1537–43.

[49] Fenner DE, Genberg B, Brahma P, et al. Fecal and urinary incontinence after vaginal delivery with anal sphincter disruption in an obstetrics unit in the United States. Am J Obstet Gynecol 2003;189:1543–9.

[50] Pollack J, Nordenstam J, Brismar S, et al. Anal incontinence after vaginal delivery: a five-year prospective cohort study. Obstet Gynecol 2004;104: 1397–402.

[51] Sultan AH, Kamm MA, Hudson CN, et al. Third degree obstetric anal sphincter tears: risk factors and outcomes of primary repair. BMJ 1994;308: 887–90.

[52] Faltin DL, Boulvain M, Floris LA, et al. Diagnosis of anal sphincter tears to prevent fecal incontinence: a randomized controlled trial. Obstet Gynecol 2005; 106:6–13.

[53] Carroli G, Belizan J. Episiotomy for vaginal birth. Cochrane Database Syst Rev 2000;(2):CD000081.

[54] Johanson RB, Menon BKV. Vacuum extraction versus forceps for assisted vaginal delivery. Cochrane Database Syst Rev 2000;(2):CD000224.

[55] Tetzschner T, Sorensen M, Lose G, et al. Anal and urinary incontinence in women with obstetric anal sphincter rupture. Br J Obstet Gynaecol 1997; 104(6):1034–40.

[56] Lal MH, Mann C, Callender R, et al. Does cesarean delivery prevent anal incontinence? Obstet Gynecol 2003;101:305–12.

[57] van Brummen HJ, Bruinse HW, van de Pol G, et al. Defecatory symptoms during and after the first pregnancy: prevalence and associated factors. Int Urogynecol J Pelvic Floor Dysfunct 2006;17(3):224–30.

[58] Nygaard I, Rao SSC, Dawson JD. Anal incontinence after anal sphincter disruption: a 30-year retrospective cohort study. Obstet Gynecol 1997;89(6): 896–901.

[59] Boyles SH, Weber AM, Meyn L. Procedures for pelvic organ prolapse in the United States, 1979–1997. Am J Obstet Gynecol 2003;188:108–15.

[60] Norton PA, Bump RC. Epidemiology and natural history of pelvic floor dysfunction. Obstet Gynecol Clin North Am 1998;25(4):724–45.

[61] Olsen AL, Smith VJ, Bergstrom JO, et al. Epidemiology of surgically managed pelvic organ prolapse and urinary incontinence. Obstet Gyencol 1997; 89(4):501–6.

[62] Barber MD. Symptoms and outcome measures of pelvic organ prolapse. Clin Obstet Gynecol 2005; 48(3):648–61.

[63] Schaffer JI, Wai Clifford Y, Boreham M. Etiology of pelvic organ prolapse. Clin Obstet Gynecol 2005; 48(3):639–47.

[64] Mant J, Painter R, Vessey M. Epidemiology of genital prolapse: observations from the Oxford Family Planning Association study. Br J Obstet Gynaecol 1997;104(5):579–85.

[65] Lukacz ES, Lawrence JM, Contreras R, et al. Parity, mode of delivery, and pelvic floor disorders. Obstet Gynecol 2006;107(6):1253–60.

[66] Sze EHM, Sherard GB, Dolezal JM. Pregnancy, labour, delivery and pelvic organ prolapse. Obstet Gynecol 2002;100(5 pt 1):981–6.

[67] Dietz HP, Eldridge A, Grace M, et al. Does pregnancy affect pelvic organ mobility? Aust N Z J Obstet Gynaecol 2004;44(6):517–20.

[68] von Sydow K. Sexuality during pregnancy and after childbirth: a metacontent analysis of 59 studies. J Psychosom Res 1999;47(1):27–49.

[69] Hames CT. Sexual needs and interests of postpartum couples. J Obstet Gynecol Neonatal Nurs 1980;9(10):313–5.

[70] Glazener CMA. Sexual function after childbirth: women's experiences, persistent morbidity and lack of professional recognition. Br J Obstet Gynaecol 1997;104:330–5.

[71] Thompson JF, Roberts CL, Currie M, et al. Prevalence and persistence of health problems after childbirth: associations with parity and method of birth. Birth 2002;29:83–94.

[72] Macarthur AJ, Macarthur C. Incidence, severity, and determinants of perineal pain after vaginal delivery: a prospective cohort study. Am J Obstet Gynecol 2004;191:1199–204.

[73] Klein MC, Gauthier RJ, Robbins JM, et al. Relationship of episiotomy to perineal trauma and morbidity, sexual dysfunction, and pelvic floor relaxation. Am J Obstet Gynecol 1994;171:591–8.

[74] Barrett G, Peacock J, Victor CR, et al. Cesarean section and postnatal sexual health. Birth 2005;32(4): 306–11.

[75] Hicks TL, Goodall SF, Quattrone EM, et al. Postpartum sexual functioning and method of delivery: summary of the evidence. J Midwifery Womens Health 2004;49(5):430–6.

[76] National Institutes of Health State-of-the-Science Conference Statement: Cesarean delivery on maternal request March 27–29, 2006. Obstet Gynecol 2006;107(6):1386–97.

[77] Wilson PD, Herbison RM, Herbison GP. Obstetric practice and the prevalence of urinary incontinence three months after delivery. Br J Obstet Gynaecol 1996;103:154–61.

[78] Schaffer JI, Bloom SL, Casey BM, et al. A randomized trial of the effects of coached vs uncoached maternal pushing during the second stage of labor on postpartum pelvic floor structure and function. Am J Obstet Gynecol 2005;192: 692–6.

[79] DeLee JB. The prophylactic forceps operation. Am J Obstet Gynecol 1920;1:34–44.

[80] Hartmann K, Viswanathan M, Palmieri R, Gartlehner G, Thorp J Jr, Lohr KN. Outcomes of routine episiotomy: a systematic review. JAMA 2005;293: 2141–8.

ELSEVIER
SAUNDERS

Urol Clin N Am 34 (2007) 23–26

UROLOGIC
CLINICS
of North America

Urologic Radiology During Pregnancy

Kevin R. Loughlin, MD[a,b,*]

[a]Division of Urology, Brigham and Women's Hospital, 45 Francis Street, Boston, MA 02115, USA
[b]Harvard Medical School Boston, MA

Radiation risk

Ionizing radiation can result in three types of harmful effects: (1) cell death and teratogenic effects, (2) carcinogenesis, and (3) genetic effects [1]. Fetal radiation exposure has been associated with intrauterine growth retardation, microcephaly, mental retardation, and fetal demise, although these events are associated with radiation doses of greater than 10 rad, which far exceeds the radiation exposure in most urologic radiologic procedures [2]. However, childhood leukemia and other childhood malignancies have been associated with modest radiation dose exposure [3,4]. Harvey and colleagues [5] reported a retrospective study of twins born in Connecticut during a 40-year period, which examined the relationship between prenatal radiation exposure and subsequent childhood malignancy. During that time, twin gestations were diagnosed by a limited plain film. It was estimated that the fetal radiation exposure ranged from 0.16–4.0 rad, with the average dose being about 1 rad. This level of exposure approximates that of an intravenous pyelogram (IVP). The Harvey study followed the cohort throughout childhood and found a 1.6 relative risk of leukemia, a 3.2 relative risk of childhood solid tumors, and an overall relative risk of 2.4 for all childhood malignancies. Some subsequent studies have confirmed this association [6], whereas others have not [7].

Radiation exposure

It would be appropriate at this point to review the radiation exposure associated with commonly performed urologic procedures. These estimates are culled from the literature [1,2,8,9] and appear in Table 1.

Ultrasonography

Ultrasound examination does not expose the fetus to any ionizing radiation. In a pregnant patient who presents with hematuria or flank pain, an abdominal ultrasound is the screening procedure of choice. Although an abdominal ultrasound is very useful to screen for renal masses and pathology outside the urinary tract, it does have limitations in the diagnosis of urolithiasis [10].

Because of the physiologic hydronephrosis of pregnancy, a transabdominal ultrasound misses many ureteral stones. Hendricks and colleagues [11] have reported a diagnostic accuracy of less than 50% with transabdominal ultrasound in pregnant women with urolithiasis. However, other ultrasound maneuvers can increase the diagnostic accuracy of an ultrasound examination.

Color Doppler ultrasound is now commonly used by radiologists [11,12]; it can be used to help differentiate physiologic dilation from obstruction in pregnancy [13]. In addition, transvaginal ultrasound has been reported by Laing and colleagues [14] as a useful adjunct in identifying distal ureteral stones in pregnant patients. A 5.0 megahertz vaginal transducer with a 90° sector angle and a 30° off-axis beam angle is used, and the technique is straightforward.

Limited intravenous pyelogram

If an ultrasound examination does not give definitive information, many urologists will opt

* Division of Urology, Brigham and Women's Hospital, 45 Francis Street, Boston, MA 02115.
 E-mail address: kloughlin@partners.org.

Table 1
Estimated exposure of urologic diagnostic procedures

Procedure	Rad
Ultrasound	0.00
MRI	0.00
CXR	0.02
KUB	0.05
Limited IVP (3–4 films)	0.20–0.25
Standard IVP	0.40–0.50
Fluoroscopy	1.50–2.00/m
CT abdomen/pelvis	2.00–2.50

Abbreviations: CXR, chest x-ray; KUB, kidneys, ureter, bladder (plain abdominal radiograph).

for a "limited" IVP, which normally includes three to four films [2]. Such a study typically delivers about 0.20–0.25 rad to the fetus.

CT

CT is ordered by some urologists if the screening ultrasound suggests a renal mass. However, the CT scan exposes the fetus to 2.0. to 2.5 rad, and in most cases of urologic pathology is an

unnecessary diagnostic test in pregnancy [15,16]. Rarely should CT scans be required to evaluate urologic problems in pregnancy.

MRI

MRI is an attractive diagnostic tool during pregnancy because it exposes the fetus to no radiation. MRI is quite sensitive in detecting hydronephrosis and the level of obstruction [17,18], but it does not visualize stones well in most cases [19]. Therefore, its use in the pregnant patient who has renal colic is limited, but it is a worthwhile second-line study after a renal mass has been detected on ultrasound.

Retrograde pyelogram/fluoroscopy

Fluoroscopy can result in considerable radiation exposure to the fetus. It is estimated that fluoroscopy results in 1.5–2.0 rad/minute. Therefore, it would appear reasonable to limit fluoroscopy during ureteroscopy and ureteral stent placement in the pregnant patient. The author and others have used intraoperative ultrasound

---

Box 1. American College of Obstetrics and Gynecology guidelines for diagnostic imaging during pregnancy

1. Women should be counseled that radiograph exposure from a single diagnostic procedure does not result in harmful fetal effects. Specifically, exposure to less than 5 rad has not been associated with an increase in fetal anomalies or pregnancy loss.[1]
2. Concern about possible effects of high-dose ionizing radiation exposure should not prevent medically indicated diagnostic radiography procedures from being performed on a pregnant woman. During pregnancy, other imaging procedures not associated with ionizing radiation (eg, ultrasonography, MRI) should be considered instead of radiographs, when appropriate.
3. Ultrasonography and MRI are not associated with known adverse fetal effects.
4. Consultation with an expert in dosimetry calculation may be helpful in calculating estimated fetal dose when multiple diagnostic radiographs are performed on a pregnant patient.
5. The use of radioactive isotopes of iodine is contraindicated for therapeutic use during pregnancy.
6. Radiopaque and paramagnetic contrast agents are unlikely to cause harm and may be of diagnostic benefit, but these agents should be used during pregnancy only if the potential benefit justifies the potential risk to the fetus.

---

[1] The last statement applies to fetal anomalies or pregnancy loss. Exposure to lower doses (0.16–4.0 rad) may be associated with increased incidence of childhood malignancies, as described in the section on radiation risk.
Adapted from American College of Obstetrics and Gynecology Committee on Obstetric Practice. ACOG Committee Opinion. Number 299, September 2004 (replaces No. 158, September 1995). Guidelines for diagnostic imaging during pregnancy. Obstet Gynecol 2004 Sep;104(3):647-51.

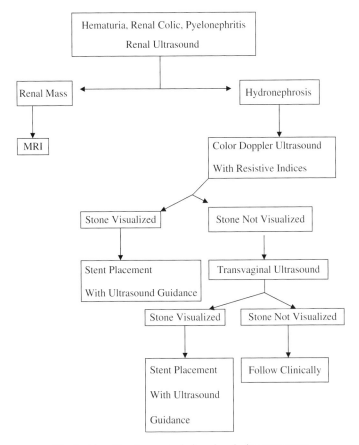

Fig. 1. Algorithm for urologic imaging during pregnancy.

[20,21] to confirm successful stent placement in these patients, and have performed ureteroscopy without the use of fluoroscopy. The need for fluoroscopy is one of the reasons that the author personally feels that percutaneous lithotripsy is not an attractive option for stone management during pregnancy [22].

Nuclear medicine

Nuclear medicine scans are performed by "tagging" a chemical agent with a radioisotope. The fetal radiation exposure is generally small, but depends on the physical and biochemical properties of the radioisotope [23]. However, radioactive iodine readily crosses the placenta and can affect the fetal thyroid, particularly if used after 10 to 12 weeks of gestation [1].

The American College of Obstetrics and Gynecology has issued guidelines for diagnostic imaging during pregnancy [1]. These guidelines appear in Box 1.

Based on the information reviewed above, the author has proposed an algorithm for the use of diagnostic imaging for urologic symptoms during pregnancy. This algorithm appears in Fig. 1.

Summary

The management of the pregnant patient who has urologic symptoms presents unique challenges. However, with the exercise of good clinical judgment and the use of the armamentarium of diagnostic imaging modalities available, the pregnant patient can be managed with minimal, if any, radiation exposure to the fetus.

References

[1] ACOG Committee on Obstetric Practice. ACOG Committee Opinion, Number 299. Guidelines For Diagnostic Imaging During Pregnancy. Obstet Gynecol 2004;104(3):647–51.
[2] Riddell JVB, Densted JD. Management of urolithiasis during pregnancy. Contemp Urol 2000;12–26.

[3] Naumburg E, Bellocco R, Cnattingius S , et al. Intra-uterine exposure to diagnostic x-rays and risk of childhood leukemia subtypes. Radiat Res 2001;156:718–23.

[4] Kusama T, Ota K. Radiological protection for diagnostic examination of pregnant women. Congenit Anom (Kyoto) 2002;42:10–4.

[5] Harvey EB, Boice JD, Honeyman JM, et al. Prenatal x-ray exposure and childhood cancer in twins. N Engl J Med 1985;312:541–5.

[6] Doll R, Wakeford R. Risk of childhood cancer from fetal irradiation. Br J Radiol 1997;70:130–9.

[7] Meinert R, Kaletsch U, Kaatsch P, et al. Associations between childhood cancer and ionizing radiation: results of a population based case control study in Germany. Cancer Epidemiol Biomarkers Prev 1999;8:793–9.

[8] Evans HJ, Wollin TA. The management of urinary calculi in pregnancy. Curr Opin Urol 2001;11(4):379–84.

[9] Wesley WM, Klein FA, Loughlin KR. Guidelines and evolving strategies in the management of urinary stone disease during pregnancy. Contemp Urol 2006;181(6):34–43.

[10] Loughlin KR, Kerr LA. The current management of urolithiasis during pregnancy. Urol Clin North Amer 2002;29:701–4.

[11] Platt JF, Rubin JM, Ellis JH, et al. Duplex Doppler US of the kidney: differentiation of obstructive from nonobstructive dilation. Radiology 1989;171:515–7.

[12] Platt JF, Rubin JM, Ellis JH. Acute renal obstruction evaluation with intrarenal Doppler and conventional US. Radiology 1993;186:685–8.

[13] Hertzberg BS, Carroll BA, Bowie JD, et al. Doppler US assessment of maternal kidneys: analysis of intrarenal resistivity indexes in normal pregnancy and physiologic pelvicaliectasis. Radiology 1993; 186:689–92.

[14] Laing FC, Benson CB, DiSalvo DN, et al. Distal ureteral calculi detection with vaginal US. Radiology 1994;192(2):545–8.

[15] Kusama T, Ota K. Radiologic protection for diagnostic examination of pregnant women. Congenit Anom (Kyoto) 2002;42:10–4.

[16] Swanson SK, Heilman RC, Everson WGH. Urinary tract stones in pregnancy. Surg Clin North Am 1995; 75:123–42.

[17] Roy C, Saussine C, Le Brad Y, et al. Assessment of painful ureterohydronephrosis during pregnancy by MR urography. Eur Radiol 1996;6:334–8.

[18] Grenier N, Pariente JL, Trillaud H, et al. Dilation of the collecting system during pregnancy: physiologic vs obstructive dilation. Eur Radiol 2000;10(2):271–9.

[19] Stoller ML, Floth A, Hricale H. Magnetic resonance imaging of renal calculi: an in vitro study. J Lithotr Stone Dis 1991;3:162–4.

[20] Gluck CD, Benson CB, Bowdy AC, et al. Renal sonograph for placement and monitoring of ureteral stents during pregnancy. J Endourol 1991;5:241–3.

[21] Jarrard DJ, Geber GS, Lyon ES. Management of acute ureteral obstruction in pregnancy utilizing ultrasound-guided placement of ureteral stents. Urol 1993;42:263–8.

[22] Kavoussi LR, Albala DM, Bosler JW, et al. Percutaneous management of urolithiasis during pregnancy. J Urol 1992;148:1069–71.

[23] Cunningham FG, Gant NF, Leveno KJ, et al. General consideration and maternal evaluation. In: Williams Obstetrics. 21st edition. New York: McGraw-Hill; 2001. p. 1143–58.

ELSEVIER
SAUNDERS

Urol Clin N Am 34 (2007) 27–33

**UROLOGIC
CLINICS
of North America**

Pharmaceutical Agents and Pregnancy in Urology Practice

Alon Shrim, MD[a], Facundo Garcia-Bournissen, MD[a],
Gideon Koren, MD[a,b],*

[a]The Motherisk Program, Division of Clinical Pharmacology/Toxicology, Hospital for Sick Children,
The University of Toronto, 555 University Avenue, Toronto, Ontario, Canada M5G 1X8
[b]Department of Paediatrics, The University of Western Ontario, 800 Commissioners Road East, Room E6-103 London,
Ontario, Canada N6A 5W9

Most drugs are not tested on pregnant women before marketing to determine their effects on the fetus. As a consequence, most of them are not labeled for use during pregnancy. Typically, descriptions of drugs that appear in the *Physician's Desk Reference* and similar sources contain statements such as "Use in pregnancy is not recommended unless the potential benefits justify the potential risks to the fetus." Because the actual risk has been adequately established for only a few drugs, physicians caring for pregnant

women have little information to help them decide whether the potential benefits to the mother outweigh the risks to the fetus.

These typical disclaimers, although understandable from the medico-legal standpoint, put large numbers of women and their physicians in difficult situations for several reasons. One is that at least half the pregnancies in North America are unplanned [1]; hence, every year hundreds of thousands of women expose their fetuses to drugs before they know they have conceived. Such women often interpret the statement that use during pregnancy is not recommended as meaning that the drug is not safe in this period. This perception of fetal risk causes many women to consider seeking or even to seek termination of otherwise wanted pregnancies. Another cause of difficulty is that, given the recent increase in the age at which women start families, large numbers of women have conditions that necessitate long-term drug therapy. Furthermore, for certain conditions once believed to be incompatible with pregnancy, such as systemic lupus erythematosus and renal transplant, the outcome of pregnancy has improved dramatically in the past few decades.

Although urologic medical conditions are not frequently encountered during pregnancy, urologists often are asked to treat pregnant patients for conditions that require prescriptions. In the generally healthy population of pregnant women, the use of pharmaceutical agents is limited and is usually reserved for women who have infections (simple or complex) or necessary surgical procedures [2].

Supported by grants from the Canadian Institute for Health Research and by the Research Leadership for Better Pharmacotherapy During Pregnancy and Lactation. Dr. Shrim is supported by the Research Training Centre, The Hospital for Sick Children, Toronto, Ontario, Canada. Dr. Garcia Bournissen is supported by the Clinician Scientist Training Program, The Hospital for Sick Children, Toronto, Ontario, Canada.

Editor's note: This article describes a 10-day course of nitrofurantoin as a common treatment for asymptomatic bacteriuria in pregnancy. Other options are described in the article on urinary tract infections in pregnancy by Macejko and Schaeffer, also in this issue. The United States Food and Drug Administration has established a five-category classification system to describe the use of drugs in pregnancy, as shown in Table 1.

* Corresponding author. Division of Clinical Pharmacology/Toxicology, Hospital for Sick Children, 555 University Avenue, Toronto, Ontario, Canada M5G 1X8.

E-mail address: gideon.koren@sickkids.ca
(G. Koren).

0094-0143/07/$ - see front matter © 2006 Elsevier Inc. All rights reserved.
doi:10.1016/j.ucl.2006.10.004

Table 1
United States Food and Drug Administration Five-category classification system

Category	Description
A	Adequate, well-controlled studies in pregnant women have not shown an increased risk of fetal abnormalities.
B	Animal studies have revealed no evidence of harm to the fetus; however, there are no adequate and well-controlled studies in pregnant women.
	or
	Animal studies have shown an adverse effect, but adequate and well-controlled studies in pregnant women have failed to demonstrate a risk to the fetus.
C	Animal studies have shown an adverse effect, and there are no adequate and well-controlled studies in pregnant women.
	or
	No animal studies have been conducted, and there are no adequate and well-controlled studies in pregnant women.
D	Studies, adequate, well-controlled, or observational, in pregnant women have demonstrated a risk to the fetus. However, the benefits of therapy may outweigh the potential risk.
X	Studies, adequate, well-controlled, or observational, in animals or pregnant women have demonstrated positive evidence of fetal abnormalities. The use of the product is contraindicated in women who are or may become pregnant.

Asymptomatic bacteriuria affects 5% to 8% of pregnant women and is typically present at the time of the first prenatal visit. If left untreated, about 25% of affected women subsequently develop acute symptomatic infection during pregnancy. Nitrofurantoin treatment for this indication is common and usually effective [3].

In light of the increasing levels of resistance of many micropathogens to the antibiotics commonly prescribed during pregnancy, the clinical use of fluoroquinolones has been increasing substantially, especially in complex infections. Their safety is an increasing concern.

Finally, pregnant women who have various conditions may require nonobstetric surgical intervention. For example, urinary stones, although more common in men than in women, have an average age of onset in the third decade; hence pregnant women are a highly susceptible population [3]. Approximately 50% of pregnant women who have symptomatic stones have associated infection, and vigorous antibacterial treatment is often indicated. In addition, one third of women who have renal stones require an invasive procedure, such as urethral stenting, percutaneous nephrostomy, laser lithotripsy, basket extraction, or, occasionally, surgical exploration [4,5].

This article addresses the implications for pregnancy of these three most common urologic

events in generally healthy pregnant women, namely simple urinary tract infections that often respond to nitrofurantoin; complex urinary tract infections that require other antibiotics, possibly including fluoroquinolones; and nonobstetric surgical intervention.

Nitrofurantoin

Nitrofurantoin is an oral antibiotic with a short elimination half-life that reaches very high concentrations in urine. It is effective against most strains of *Escherichia coli* and gram-positive and gram-negative urinary tract pathogens, except for most strains of *Klebsiella, Enterobacter, Pseudomonas,* and *Proteus*, against which it has limited activity.

Nitrofurantoin is effective in asymptomatic bacteriuria and uncomplicated cystitis in women. It may also be used as prophylaxis to prevent recurrent bacteriuria after an episode of urinary tract infection, once the infection has been adequately treated [6]. Nitrofurantoin is an interesting alternative to other antibiotics, such as beta-lactams and trimethoprim-sulfamethoxazole (TMS), given the high rates of resistance of *E coli* in many geographic areas and concerns about adverse effects on the fetus and newborn with use of TMS (eg, increased neural tube defects and kernicterus) [7]. Resistance to nitrofurantoin appears to remain low in most regions [6].

Nitrofurantoin has not been linked to congenital malformations in humans or in animal studies using doses as great as 50 times the human dose [8,9]. Human case series and case control studies have failed to show an association between nitrofurantoin use during pregnancy and malformations in the newborns [10–12]. A meta-analysis including most published evidence on nitrofurantoin use during pregnancy also found no association between its usage and malformations [13].

A theoretic risk for hemolytic anemia exists in newborns exposed perinatally to nitrofurantoin, because of immaturity of erythrocyte enzyme systems; this is a particular concern in neonates who have glucose-6-phosphate dehydrogenase deficiency. Despite the paucity of published evidence for this potential complication, nitrofurantoin use is still discouraged near term (37 to 42 weeks of gestation) and during labor and delivery [6,14,15].

Fluoroquinolones

As often happens in research of drug effects on the fetus, fluoroquinolones (FQs) represent an interesting paradigm of contrasting data in animal and human studies.

Since their introduction in the 1960s with nalidixic acid, quinolone antimicrobial agents have undergone substantial development, resulting in improved antimicrobial activity, pharmacokinetic features, and toxicity profiles. The most important breakthrough, however, was the development of FQs in the 1980s, with their broad antibacterial spectra, excellent pharmacologic properties, and low incidence of serious adverse effects [16].

FQs are used widely in clinical practice as treatment for urinary infections, urogenital infections, and sexually transmitted diseases [17]. In addition, despite some continuing controversy, an increasing number of clinicians support the use of prophylactic antibacterial agents in various urologic procedures, such as urethral catheterization, endoscopy of the urinary tract, transurethral surgery, and selected open urologic procedures [18].

In parallel, teratogenic and fetotoxic concerns have been raised regarding the use of fluoroquinolones during pregnancy. Mammalian DNA shares similar topoisomerases with micropathogens. Given this factor and the ability of fluoroquinolones to cross the animal and human placenta

[19,20], they can theoretically have mutagenic effects on the developing fetus. Furthermore, the quinolones have a high affinity to cartilage: studies in beagle dogs and guinea pigs have demonstrated fetal arthropathy of weight-bearing joints after the administration of 30 mg/kg and 90 mg/kg of ciprofloxacin [21]. Similar histopathologic changes of the principal weight-bearing joints (chondrocyte loss, matrix degeneration, and erosion of the articular cartilage) were reported in fetal mice treated with quinolones [22]. Adding to the high index of suspicion of teratogenicity are arthralgia and tendonitis that have been rarely reported in adolescents and adults treated with this compound [23,24]. Eventually, the use of these drugs in children and pregnant women was restricted, particularly based on the toxicity observed in immature animals.

The available human data regarding the safety of FQ use during pregnancy are based primarily on three substantial studies. The first study [25] focused on the musculoskeletal system: 38 pregnant women who received quinolones were tested for perinatal complications, birth weights, birth defects, and developmental milestones. They were compared with controls, matched for both maternal age and indication for antibacterial therapy. Thirty-five women (92%) received therapy during the first trimester, primarily for urinary tract infection. Children born to mothers treated with quinolones were significantly heavier and had a higher rate of cesarean section than the control infants. However, no malformations were found in the quinolone group, whereas one child in the control group had a ventricular septal defect. No differences were detected between the groups in achievement of developmental milestones or in the musculoskeletal system.

An additional study, conducted 2 years later [17], was a prospective follow-up of pregnant women who contacted a teratology information center for risk information on FQ treatment. A total of 549 pregnancies were collected and followed up. No specific patterns of congenital abnormalities were found. The results did not suggest an elevated risk for spontaneous abortions, prematurity, intrauterine growth retardation, postnatal disorders, or malformations.

A more recent study [26] was designed to examine whether in utero exposure to FQs is associated with clinically significant musculoskeletal dysfunctions. Two hundred women exposed to FQs during gestation were prospectively enrolled and followed up; 136 of them were exposed during the first trimester (organogenesis period). Pregnancy outcome was compared with that of 200 controls who were exposed to nonteratogenic, nonembryotoxic antimicrobial agents and who were matched by indication, duration of therapy, trimester of exposure, age, smoking, and alcohol consumption. Rates of major or minor congenital malformations did not differ between the groups. Women treated with FQs tended to have an increased rate of therapeutic abortions compared with the rate among women exposed to nonteratogens, resulting in lower live-birth rates. The rates of spontaneous abortions, fetal distress, prematurity, and low birth weight did not differ between the groups. Here again, no clinically significant musculoskeletal dysfunctions were noted in children exposed to FQs in utero.

Analyzing the current data, it appears that, in the case of FQs, animal data suggestive of damage to weight-bearing joints may not be related to potential human risks. Importantly, human babies do not stand until the age of 1 year and hence do not bear weight. In the era of increasing resistance of many micropathogens to various antibacterial agents, FQs should not be prescribed as routine first-line agents for the treatment of uncomplicated urinary tract infections. However, in selected cases of infections with resistant micropathogens or complicated urinary tract infections during pregnancy when the use of FQs is indicated, or in cases of inadvertent fetal exposure to FQs (unplanned pregnancies), it appears that the risks to the human fetus are unproven and are generally outweighed by the benefits of FQs.

Surgery and general anesthesia

Surgery during pregnancy is an uncommon event but one that creates a great deal of anxiety for both patients and practitioners. It has been estimated that between 0.5% and 2.2% of pregnant women undergo surgical procedures unrelated to an obstetric indication [27,28]. Laparoscopy is the most commonly performed first-trimester intervention (most commonly for ectopic pregnancies), and appendectomy is the most common procedure during the remainder of the pregnancy [29,30]. Delay in diagnosis and treatment, secondary to pregnancy, may interfere with the diagnosis when reporting high maternal and fetal morbidity.

The risk for an adverse pregnancy outcome does not appear to be increased in women who undergo most uncomplicated, minor surgical procedures [3]. This is not the case when a major inflammation or infection process is involved. In this regard, appendicitis in pregnancy has been well studied; perforated appendicitis with purulent peritonitis is associated with significant maternal and fetal morbidity and mortality, even when the surgical and anesthetic techniques are flawless [3]. In contrast, procedure-related complications may adversely affect pregnancy outcome independently of their initial cause. An example would be the case of a woman who has uncomplicated removal of an inflamed appendix and may suffer aspiration of acidic gastric contents on extubation.

The Swedish Birth Registry [29] studied the effects of 5405 nonobstetric surgical procedures performed in pregnant women from 1973 to 1981. Sixty percent of the procedures were abdominal or pelvic, 20% were gynecologic and urologic, and 15% were laparoscopic procedures. In more than half of the procedures, general anesthesia was administered, mostly with nitrous oxide supplemented by another inhalation agent or intravenous medications. Maternal and fetal outcomes were compared with those of 720,000 pregnancies without antepartum surgery. Rates of stillbirths and congenital malformations were similar in the two groups, a result that is consistent with other reports. However, there was a significantly increased incidence of low birth weights and preterm births, as well as of neonatal deaths, in women who had undergone surgery.

Stepp and colleagues [31] analyzed pregnancy outcomes following abdominal surgery. An adverse outcome was defined as delivery within 14 days of surgery, delivery of a nonviable fetus, or preterm delivery at less than 37 weeks of gestation. Two factors were found in this study to be associated with adverse outcome: peritonitis and procedure length. These results may imply that the primary medical condition (ie, the cause of the intervention) is more predictive of the pregnancy outcome than is the surgery per se.

Czeizel and colleagues [32] examined the effect of anesthetic agents in pregnancy in the large population-based data set of the Hungarian Case-Control Surveillance of Congenital Abnormalities. Comparing more than 40,000 women, they found no increased risk for malformations in women who underwent surgery during pregnancy. A lower birth weight was found in healthy newborn infants born to mothers who had surgery during pregnancy; however, this could be attributed to a subgroup who had cervical incompetence—often treated with cerclage, which is of limited efficacy. This study challenges an earlier study by Kallen and Mazze [33], who suggested a possible causal relationship with neural-tube defects in 572 women who had operations at 4 to 5 weeks of gestation.

A recent systematic review by the Motherisk program has evaluated the effect of nonobstetric surgical procedures on pregnancy outcome [34]. Fifty-four articles describing 4473 patients matched the inclusion criteria for the systematic review. Only one maternal death of a woman undergoing laparoscopic cholecystectomy due to intra-abdominal hemorrhage has been reported, corresponding to a maternal death rate of 0.006%. The overall number of reported miscarriages was 236, corresponding to 5.8% of all reported patients. Even though this figure is not high, it cannot be evaluated in the absence of a control group. The rate of delivery induced by surgical intervention was 3.5%, and such delivery was most prevalent in women who had appendectomy in pregnancy. A total of 2.5% of pregnancies resulted in fetal loss, and the rate of prematurity was 8.2%. The rate of malformations was 2% and was highest in patients who underwent surgical procedures during the first trimester (3.9%). Notably, appendectomy during pregnancy carried an apparently higher risk for surgery-induced delivery (4.6%) and fetal loss (2.6% without peritonitis and 10.9% with peritonitis, versus 1.2% in surgeries for other indications).

Over the past decade, the use of laparoscopic techniques has become extremely common for diagnosis and management of a number of surgical disorders complicating pregnancy. Lachman and colleagues [35] reviewed 518 laparoscopic procedures performed during pregnancy (45% cholecystectomy, 34% adnexal surgery, 15% appendectomy, and 6% other operations). They reported similar hemodynamic changes induced by abdominal insufflation for laparoscopy in pregnant and nonpregnant women. Steinbrook and Bhavani-Shankar [36] used noninvasive hemodynamic monitoring in four healthy women at 17 to 24 weeks during scheduled laparoscopic cholecystectomy. Compared with preinduction values, the mean arterial pressures, systemic vascular resistance, and heart rate did not change significantly and were similar to those reported in nonpregnant women [37].

The precise effects of laparoscopy on the human fetus are unknown. To study the impact of laparoscopy on perinatal outcomes, Reedy and colleagues [38] used the Swedish Birth Registry. Between 1973 and 1993, there were slightly more than 2 million deliveries. There were 2181 laparoscopies and 1522 laparotomies performed in these women. Laparoscopy was performed primarily during the first trimester. Perinatal outcomes in women undergoing surgery were compared with those of all women in the database. The investigators confirmed previous studies and found an increased risk for low birth weight, preterm delivery, and fetal growth restriction in the operative group. No differences were found in malformation rates or perinatal outcome when laparoscopy and laparotomy were compared.

In a more recent nationwide, multicenter retrospective study, including 17 hospitals throughout Israel [39], the outcome of pregnancy in 389 pregnant women who had laparoscopy or laparotomy was reported. In 192 laparoscopies and 197 laparotomies performed, 6 and 25 women had complications, respectively. No significant difference was found in abortion rates, mean gestational ages at delivery, or mean birth weights between the groups. No significant difference was found in frequency of fetal anomalies between the groups or when they were compared with the national registry of anomalies. Overall, the existing data suggest that reproductive risks associated with laparoscopy are probably not increased during pregnancy.

Summary

Many pregnant women require drug therapy because of pregnancy-induced conditions. As a general rule, because fetal safety is a major concern, effective drugs that have been in use for long periods are preferable to new, less studied alternatives. To minimize fetal risk, drug doses at the lower end of the therapeutic range should be prescribed first during pregnancy, and doses should be increased only when clinically needed. Over-the-counter drugs should not be taken without counseling, because many factors, including the stage of pregnancy, can influence the risk to the fetus. In addition to the risk associated with fetal exposure to teratogenic drugs, there is a risk associated with misinformation regarding the teratogenicity of drugs, which can lead to unnecessary abortions or the avoidance of needed therapy. Health care providers should make a concerted effort to protect women and their unborn babies from both risks.

References

[1] Sophocles AM Jr, Brozovich EM. Birth control failure among patients with unwanted pregnancies: 1982–1984. J Fam Pract 1986;22(1):45–8.

[2] Suchanek P, Nagy V, Lukacin S. [Effect of acute urological complications on the course of pregnancy.] Ceska Gynekol 2003;68(5):336–40.

[3] Leveno KJ, Cunningham FG, Grant NF. William's Obstetrics. 22nd edition. Columbus (OH): McGraw-Hill; 2005.

[4] Butler EL, Cox SM, Eberts EG, et al. Symptomatic nephrolithiasis complicating pregnancy. Obstet Gynecol 2000;96(5 Pt 1):753–6.

[5] Lewis DF, Robichaux AG III, Jaekle RK, et al. Urolithiasis in pregnancy. Diagnosis, management and pregnancy outcome. J Reprod Med 2003;48(1):28–32.

[6] Le J, Briggs GG, McKeown A, et al. Urinary tract infections during pregnancy. Ann Pharmacother 2004;38(10):1692–701.

[7] Mazzulli T. Resistance trends in urinary tract pathogens and impact on management. J Urol 2002;168(4 Pt 2):1720–2.

[8] Procter & Gamble Pharmaceuticals. Macrodantin: product monograph. Cinncinnati (OH): Procter & Gamble Pharmaceuticals 2001.

[9] Briggs GG. Drugs in pregnancy and lactation. 7th edition. Philadelphia: Lippincott, Williams & Wilkins; 2005.

[10] Czeizel AE, Rockenbauer M, Sorensen HT, et al. Nitrofurantoin and congenital abnormalities. Eur J Obstet Gynecol Reprod Biol 2001;95(1):119–26.

[11] Hailey FJ, Fort H, Williams JC, et al. Foetal safety of nitrofurantoin macrocrystals therapy during pregnancy: a retrospective analysis. J Int Med Res 1983;11(6):364–9.

[12] Lenke RR, VanDorsten JP, Schifrin BS. Pyelonephritis in pregnancy: a prospective randomized trial to prevent recurrent disease evaluating suppressive therapy with nitrofurantoin and close surveillance. Am J Obstet Gynecol 1983;146(8):953–7.

[13] Ben DS, Einarson T, Ben DY, et al. The safety of nitrofurantoin during the first trimester of pregnancy: meta-analysis. Fundam Clin Pharmacol 1995;9(5):503–7.

[14] Bruel H, Guillemant V, Saladin-Thiron C, et al. [Hemolytic anemia in a newborn after maternal treatment with nitrofurantoin at the end of pregnancy.] Arch Pediatr 2000;7(7):745–7.

[15] Gait JE. Hemolytic reactions to nitrofurantoin in patients with glucose-6-phosphate dehydrogenase deficiency: theory and practice. DICP 1990;24(12):1210–3.

[16] Lipsky BA, Baker CA. Fluoroquinolone toxicity profiles: a review focusing on newer agents. Clin Infect Dis 1999;28(2):352–64.

[17] Schaefer C, Moura-Elefant E, Vial T, et al. Pregnancy outcome after prenatal quinolone exposure. Evaluation of a case registry of the European Network of Teratology Information Services (ENTIS). Eur J Obstet Gynecol Reprod Biol 1996;69(2):83–9.

[18] Amin M. Antibacterial prophylaxis in urology: a review. Am J Med 1992;92(4A):114S–7S.

[19] Giamarellou H, Kolokythas E, Petrikkos G, et al. Pharmacokinetics of three newer quinolones in pregnant and lactating women. Am J Med 1989;87(5A):49S–51S.

[20] Aramayona JJ, Garcia MA, Fraile LJ, et al. Placental transfer of enrofloxacin and ciprofloxacin in rabbits. Am J Vet Res 1994;55(9):1313–8.

[21] von Keutz E, Ruhl-Fehlert C, Drommer W, et al. Effects of ciprofloxacin on joint cartilage in immature dogs immediately after dosing and after a 5-month treatment-free period. Arch Toxicol 2004;78(7):418–24.

[22] Linseman DA, Hampton LA, Branstetter DG. Quinolone-induced arthropathy in the neonatal mouse. Morphological analysis of articular lesions produced by pipemidic acid and ciprofloxacin. Fundam Appl Toxicol 1995;28(1):59–64.

[23] Alfaham M, Holt ME, Goodchild MC. Arthropathy in a patient with cystic fibrosis taking ciprofloxacin. Br Med J (Clin Res Ed) 1987;295(6600):699.

[24] Schacht P, Arcieri G, Hullmann R. Safety of oral ciprofloxacin. An update based on clinical trial results. Am J Med 1989;87(5A):98S–102S.

[25] Berkovitch M, Pastuszak A, Gazarian M, et al. Safety of the new quinolones in pregnancy. Obstet Gynecol 1994;84(4):535–8.

[26] Loebstein R, Addis A, Ho E, et al. Pregnancy outcome following gestational exposure to fluoroquinolones: a multicenter prospective controlled study. Antimicrob Agents Chemother 1998;42(6):1336–9.

[27] Brodsky JB, Cohen EN, Brown BW Jr, et al. Surgery during pregnancy and fetal outcome. Am J Obstet Gynecol 1980;138(8):1165–7.

[28] Jenkins TM, Mackey SF, Benzoni EM, et al. Nonobstetric surgery during gestation: risk factors for lower birthweight. Aust N Z J Obstet Gynaecol 2003;43(1):27–31.

[29] Mazze RI, Kallen B. Reproductive outcome after anesthesia and operation during pregnancy: a registry study of 5405 cases. Am J Obstet Gynecol 1989;161(5):1178–85.

[30] Kuczkowski KM. The safety of anaesthetics in pregnant women. Expert Opin Drug Saf 2006;5(2):251–64.

[31] Stepp KJ, Sauchak, O'Malley DM, et al. Risk factors for adverse outcomes after intraabdominal surgery during pregnancy. Obstet Gynecol 2002;99:23S.

[32] Czeizel AE, Pataki T, Rockenbauer M. Reproductive outcome after exposure to surgery under anesthesia during pregnancy. Arch Gynecol Obstet 1998;261(4):193–9.

[33] Kallen B, Mazze RI. Neural tube defects and first trimester operations. Teratology 1990;41(6):717–20.

[34] Cohen-Kerem R, Railton C, Oren D, et al. Pregnancy outcome following non-obstetric surgical intervention. Am J Surg 2005;190(3):467–73.

[35] Lachman E, Schienfeld A, Voss E, et al. Pregnancy and laparoscopic surgery. J Am Assoc Gynecol Laparosc 1999;6(3):347–51.

[36] Steinbrook RA, Bhavani-Shankar K. Hemodynamics during laparoscopic surgery in pregnancy. Anesth Analg 2001;93(6):1570–1.

[37] Wahba RW, Beique F, Kleiman SJ. Cardiopulmonary function and laparoscopic cholecystectomy. Can J Anaesth 1995;42(1):51–63.

[38] Reedy MB, Kallen B, Kuehl TJ. Laparoscopy during pregnancy: a study of five fetal outcome parameters with use of the Swedish Health Registry. Am J Obstet Gynecol 1997;177(3):673–9.

[39] Oelsner G, Stockheim D, Soriano D, et al. Pregnancy outcome after laparoscopy or laparotomy in pregnancy. J Am Assoc Gynecol Laparosc 2003;10(2):200–4.

ELSEVIER
SAUNDERS

Urol Clin N Am 34 (2007) 35–42

UROLOGIC
CLINICS
of North America

Asymptomatic Bacteriuria and Symptomatic Urinary Tract Infections During Pregnancy

Amanda M. Macejko, MD, Anthony J. Schaeffer, MD*

Department of Urology, Northwestern University, 303 East Chicago Avenue, Tarry 16-703, Chicago, IL 60611, USA

Urinary tract infections (UTIs), a common complication of pregnancy, may be classified as lower (cystitis and asymptomatic bacteriuria [ASB]) or upper (pyelonephritis) tract infections. Although the prevalence of cystitis and ASB are similar in pregnant and nonpregnant women, lower tract UTIs represent a significant risk factor for developing pyelonephritis in pregnant women [1]. The increased risk of pyelonephritis is thought to be secondary to the anatomic and physiologic changes that occur in pregnancy [2]. Because pyelonephritis during pregnancy may cause significant morbidity for both the mother and the fetus, proper screening and treatment of bacteriuria, regardless of the presence of symptoms, is necessary to prevent complications.

Pathogenesis

In normal circumstances, the genitourinary tract is sterile. Bacteriuria occurs when bacteria from a fecal reservoir gain access to the bladder by ascending the urethra [3]. Organisms causing bacteriuria are similar in both pregnant and nonpregnant women (Box 1) [2], with *E coli* being the most common pathogen [4]. Other microorganisms, including *Gardnerella vaginalis*, lactobacilli, *Chlamydia trachomatis* and *Ureaplasma urealyticum*, have been found in urine. Although the clinical significance of these organisms is not yet appreciated, a few small studies have reported improved outcomes following therapy [5,6].

Urinary tract changes in pregnancy

Although the incidence of bacteriuria in pregnant women is similar to that in their nonpregnant counterparts, the incidence of acute pyelonephritis in pregnant women with bacteriuria is significantly increased, compared with nonpregnant women [7]. Anatomic and physiologic urinary tract changes in pregnancy may cause pregnant women with bacteriuria to have an increased susceptibility to pyelonephritis [2]. These urinary tract changes involve nearly the entire tract, including the kidneys, collecting system, ureters, and bladder (Box 2). The kidneys increase in length by approximately 1 centimeters during pregnancy [8]. With this increase in renal size, the glomerular filtration rate increases by approximately 30% to 50% [9]. This change is important to consider when dosing medications because the rate of renal excretion may be increased, thus reducing the duration a particular drug is present in the urine [10]. The renal pelvis and ureters may begin to dilate as early as the seventh week of pregnancy [2]. This dilation progresses throughout the course of the pregnancy and is secondary to mechanical obstruction caused by the uterus, and smooth muscle relaxation caused by progesterone. This smooth muscle relaxation results in decreased peristalsis of the ureters [4], increased bladder capacity, and urinary stasis. The bladder itself is displaced superiorly and anteriorly during pregnancy [8].

Antimicrobials in pregnancy

In treating pyelonephritis in pregnant women, it is important to remember that therapy must be safe for both mother and fetus. Nearly all

* Corresponding author.
E-mail address: ajschaeffer@northwestern.edu (A.J. Schaeffer).

Box 1. Microbiology of bacteriuria in pregnancy

Enterobacteriaceae (90%): E coli, Klebsiella, Enterobacter
Other Gram-negatives
- *P. mirabilis*
- *Pseudomonas*
- *Citrobacter*

Gram-positives
- *Staphylococcus saprophyticus*
- *Group B streptococcus* (GBS)

Other organisms
- *Gardnerella vaginalis*
- *Ureaplasma urealyticum*

Data from Gilstrap 3rd LC, Ramin SM. Urinary tract infections during pregnancy. Obstet Gynecol Clin North Am 2001;28(3):581–91; Millar LK, Cox SM. Urinary tract infections complicating pregnancy. Infect Dis Clin North Am 1997;11(1):13–26; Le J, Briggs GG, McKeown A, et al. Urinary tract infections during pregnancy. Ann Pharmacother 2004;38(10):1692–701.

antimicrobials cross the placenta, and therefore agents that may be harmful to the developing fetus should be avoided. Penicillins, cephalosporins, and nitrofurantoin have been used for a number of years without adverse fetal outcomes (Table 1) [11]. Drugs that should be avoided during pregnancy because of adverse fetal effects include fluoroquinolones[1], chloramphenicol, erythromycin, and tetracycline.

The treating physician must also remain aware that serum and tissue drug concentrations may be lowered because of the physiologic changes of pregnancy. These changes include increased maternal fluid volume, drug distribution to the fetus, increased renal blood flow, and increased glomerular filtration [3,11].

Penicillins

Penicillins have been used for a number of years, are mostly well tolerated, and are not

---

[1] It is generally recommended that fluoroquinolones be avoided during pregnancy, as described in this article. However, a different opinion is given by Shrim and colleagues in their article on pharmaceutical agents in pregnancy, elsewhere in this issue.

known to be teratogenic [10]. Ampicillin is given parenterally and may require an increased dose or frequency in pregnant women because it is rapidly excreted renally [12]. Ampicillin's oral counterpart, amoxicillin, does not require increased dosage and has been a mainstay of UTI treatment in pregnancy. However, increasing resistance to both ampicillin and amoxicillin has been observed, and therefore one should use susceptibility testing to guide treatment [13]. Penicillin G is effective and remains the drug of choice for group B streptococci bacteriuria [11].

Cephalosporins

Cephalosporins are also used commonly in pregnancy. These agents are a good choice for pyelonephritis, especially when there is resistance to first-line therapy [14]. Cephalexin, a first-generation cephalosporin, is the most commonly used oral cephalosporin [15]. Third-generation cephalosporins have excellent coverage against gram-negative, and some gram-positive, organisms. It is important to note however, that cephalosporins are not active against *Enterococcus* [11]. The clinician should also keep in mind that doses may need to be altered because cephalosporins may have a shorter half-life in pregnancy owing to increased renal clearance [16].

Box 2. Urinary tract changes in pregnancy

Kidneys
- Increased renal length
- Increased glomerular filtration rate by 30% to 50%

Collecting system
- Decreased peristalsis

Ureters
- Decreased peristalsis
- Mechanical obstruction

Bladder
- Displacement superiorly and anteriorly
- Smooth muscle relaxation

Data from Waltzer WC. The urinary tract in pregnancy. J Urol 1981;125(3):271–6.

Table 1
Antimicrobials in pregnancy

Drug	Fetal toxicity	Comments
Safe in pregnancy		
Penicillins		
Penicillin G		Used for GBS
Ampicillin		Increasing bacterial resistance
Amoxicillin		Increasing bacterial resistance
Cephalosporins		Not active against *Enterococcus*
Cephalexin		Used extensively
Cefaclor		Effective against gram-negatives
Clindamycin		Used for GBS in penicillin-allergic patients
Use cautiously in pregnancy		
Nitrofurantoin	3rd trimester: theoretical risk of fetal hemolytic anemia when mother has G6PD deficiency	Not effective in pyelonephritis Not active against *Proteus* Hemolytic anemia in maternal G6PD deficiency Rare maternal pulmonary reaction
Aminoglycosides	Theoretical risk of fetal oto- and nephrotoxicity	May cause maternal oto- and nephrotoxicity
Sulfisoxazole	1st trimester: antifolate metabolism associated with theoretical increased risk of neural tube defects 3rd trimester: may lead to neonatal hyperbilirubinemia with kernicterus	Increasing *E coli* resistance Hemolytic anemia in G6PD deficiency
Trimethoprim	1st trimester: antifolate metabolism associated with theoretical increased risk of neural tube defects	Increasing *E coli* resistance May cause maternal megaloblastic anemia
Avoid in pregnancy		
Fluoroquinolones	Irreversible arthropathy in animal studies	
Chloramphenicol	"Gray baby syndrome"	
Erythromycin		May cause maternal cholestasis
Tetracycline	Discoloration of deciduous teeth	May cause maternal acute fatty liver degeneration

Abbreviation: G6PD, glucose-6-phosphare dehydrogenase.

Data from Schaeffer AJ. Infections of the urinary tract. In: Walsh PC, Retik AB, Vaughan ED Jr, editors. Campbell's Urology. 8th edition. Philadelphia: WB Saunders; 2002. p. 516–602; Dashe JS, Gilstrap 3rd LC. Antibiotic use in pregnancy. Obstet Gynecol Clin North Am 1997;24(3):617–29.

Nitrofurantoin

Nitrofurantoin attains therapeutic levels in urine and is an acceptable agent for ASB or cystitis; however, it does not achieve adequate tissue penetration, and therefore should not be used in pyelonephritis. Nitrofurantoin is a good choice for penicillin-allergic patients or for those with resistant organisms, but it is not active against *Proteus* sp [10]. Rare, but serious, complications of nitrofurantoin include pneumonitis or pulmonary reaction and hemolytic anemia in mothers with glucose-6-phosphate dehydrogenase deficiency [1]. Nitrofurantoin has not been associated with fetal malformations [17].

Macrolides

Clindamycin is recommended for group B streptococci in pregnant women who are allergic to penicillin. It is unnecessary to increase the dose in pregnancy and teratogenicity has not been reported [18].

Aminoglycosides

This group of antimicrobials is often used in combination with ampicillin for the treatment of acute pyelonephritis during pregnancy. Aminoglycosides are particularly effective because they achieve high renal parenchymal concentrations [14]. Gentamicin is the most commonly used aminoglycoside in pregnancy. Because aminoglycosides are known to cross the placenta, they could cause ototoxicity and nephrotoxicity in the fetus [11]. However, no congenital anomalies, or ototoxicity or nephrotoxicity, after in utero exposure to aminoglycosides, have been reported [11].

Sulfonamides

This class of antimicrobials is not recommended as first-line agents because of the incidence of *E coli* resistance and toxicity. Sulfonamides may also be associated with antifolate teratogenicity in the first trimester [19]. Additionally, in the third trimester, sulfonamides can displace bilirubin from albumin, and have been reported to cause hyperbilirubinemia with kernicterus [11]. Hemolytic anemia in a fetus with a mother with glucose-6-phosphate dehydrogenase deficiency has also been reported.

Trimethoprim

Resistance of *E coli* to trimethoprim (TMP) is common, decreasing its efficacy as a first-line agent. Studies have not demonstrated teratogenicity; however, because TMP inhibits folate metabolism, theoretically it could increase the risk of neural tube defects [12]. Therefore, TMP should not be used in the first trimester [20].

Quinolones

Although quinolones achieve high concentrations within renal tissue and are appropriate for treatment of pyelonephritis in nonpregnant women, they are not recommended for pregnant women. Fluoroquinolones have been shown to impair cartilage development in animal studies. Although this adverse effect has not been described in humans, quinolones should be avoided in pregnancy [3].

Tetracycline

Tetracycline is not an appropriate agent to use in pregnancy because it leads to discoloration of deciduous teeth if given after 5 months' gestation [1,11]. Early reports suggested that tetracycline also caused enamel hypoplasia and inhibition of fibula growth; however, Porter and colleagues [21] have reported evidence that refutes these claims. Despite this, tetracyclines are Food and Drug Administration category D, and therefore should not be used in pregnancy. High doses of tetracycline in the treatment of pyelonephritis have also been reported to cause acute fatty liver degeneration [22].

Asymptomatic bacteriuria of pregnancy

Definition

ASB is essentially an asymptomatic UTI. In other words, it is the presence of significant bacteriuria without symptoms or signs, such as frequency, urgency, dysuria, pyuria, or hematuria. Significant bacteriuria is defined as greater than or equal to 10^5 colony-forming units of a single pathogen per milliliter of urine in two consecutive midstream urine samples [23]. Counts as low as 10^2 colony-forming units per milliliter should be considered significant bacteriuria if the specimen is catheterized urine or if the patient is symptomatic.

Epidemiology

Pregnancy itself is not a risk factor for ASB because ASB occurs in 4% to 6% of pregnant and nonpregnant women [24]. Socioeconomic status is a significant risk factor for ASB; it has been reported that indigent women have a fivefold greater incidence of bacteriuria, compared with nonindigent populations [25,26]. Other risk factors include diabetes, sickle cell disease and trait, multiparity, history of UTI, and anatomic or functional urinary tract abnormalities [1,25].

Significance

ASB is not considered clinically significant in most patient populations; however, this is not the case with pregnant women. The number of pregnant women who develop pyelonephritis is significantly higher than their nonpregnant counterparts. If untreated, as many as 20% to 40% of pregnant women with ASB will develop pyelonephritis [2,4,27]. Treatment of bacteriuria early in pregnancy has been shown to decrease the incidence of pyelonephritis by 90% [28]. Although it is known that bacteriuria can lead to pyelonephritis in pregnancy, other adverse effects of bacteriuria are less well-established. In various studies, untreated bacteriuria has been linked with prematurity, low birth weight, intrauterine growth retardation, and neonatal death [29]. However, poor outcomes may be the result of coexisting risk factors, such as low socioeconomic status, rather than of bacteriuria alone. To date, this suggestion remains controversial [2].

Group B streptococcus has been linked to premature rupture of membranes, preterm delivery, neonatal sepsis, meningitis, and pneumonia. Women with group B streptococcal bacteriuria should be treated at initial diagnosis and at the onset of labor [1].

Screening

The American College of Obstetricians and Gynecologists currently recommends screening for ASB in all pregnant women. A study of 3254 pregnant women determined that the optimal timing for bacteriuria screening was at 16 weeks gestation [4,30]. Urine culture is the gold standard, and all pregnant women should provide a urine specimen for culture during the first trimester [1]. A single voided specimen with 10^5 bacteria per milliliter of urine is 80% specific, whereas two specimens with the same organism are 95% specific for bacteriuria [23,31]. Using a single specimen to diagnose bacteriuria may lead to an overestimation because women with either contamination or transient bacteriuria will be included [32]. Therefore, a confirmatory culture is desirable for most cases of ASB. However, considering the risks of bacteriuria in pregnancy, in this setting it is appropriate to treat without the confirmatory culture.

If the initial negative urine culture is negative, repeat cultures are not recommended [33] because only 1% to 2% of women with initial negative cultures will go on to develop pyelonephritis during pregnancy [34]. Exceptions include women with a history of recurrent UTI, or those with known urinary tract abnormalities. These women should undergo follow-up urine cultures throughout the remainder of pregnancy.

Because urine cultures are expensive, efforts to find a more cost-effective method of detecting bacteriuria have been evaluated. However, these other methods fail to be as reliable as urine culture. For example, pyuria is not always present in bacteriuria, nor is it specific for bacteriuria. McNair and colleagues [35] reported a 53% false-negative rate with dipstick screening of nitrite and leukocyte esterase in pregnant patients. A cost analysis by Wadland and colleagues [36] found that screening with urine culture was cost-

effective, and it remains the recommended method of screening.

Treatment

Screening and treatment for ASB significantly decreases the risk of symptomatic UTI and its complications. Sweet [7] reported that treatment of ASB decreases the incidence of pyelonephritis during pregnancy from 13.5% to 65% down to 5.3% to zero. The duration of therapy has been a topic of debate, and treatment duration varies from a single dose to one week (Table 2). Single-dose therapy cure rates have been reported at 50% to 60% [37]. Efficacy rates of 70% to 80% have been shown following 3-day courses of antimicrobials. Cure rates do not improve with longer courses of therapy [38] and thus, 3-day therapy is recommended [2].

A follow-up culture 1 week following therapy to ensure that bacteriuria is eliminated should be obtained. In 20% to 30% of patients, short-course therapy will fail. In these cases, a repeat 7- to 10-day course with a culture-specific antimicrobial is appropriate [39].

Prevention

After a negative culture is obtained, daily antimicrobial suppression should be considered, which may consist of 50 to 100 mg of nitrofurantoin orally nightly [1,40]. Without prophylaxis, as many as one third of women will experience recurrent infections during pregnancy [2,32]. If suppression is not used following treatment of ASB, women should have frequent urine cultures throughout the remainder of pregnancy to identify recurrent bacteriuria. In women with recurrent or persistent bacteriuria, follow-up cultures should also be obtained after delivery. Additionally, a urologic evaluation 3 to 6 months postpartum is appropriate [41].

Symptomatic UTI

Lower UTI (acute cystitis)

Incidence of cystitis during pregnancy has been approximated at 1% to 2%. Diagnosis of cystitis is based on a combination of bacteriuria and signs and symptoms of frequency, urgency, dysuria, hematuria, and pyuria. Treatment of cystitis is the same as treatment for ASB (see Table 2). Again, follow-up as outlined above is important because up to one third of women may experience recurrent UTI during pregnancy [1].

Table 2
Treatment regimens for ASB and cystitis

Antimicrobial	Single-dose regimens	Short-course regimens
Amoxicillin	3 g OR	250–500 mg tid × 3 or 7 d
	2 g + 1 g probenecid	3 g × two doses 12 h apart
Amoxicillin/clavulanic acid	–	250/125 tid × 7 d
Nitrofurantoin	200 mg	100 mg qid × 3 or 7 d
Sulfisoxazole	2 g	1 g then 500 mg qid × 7 d
Cephalexin	2–3 g OR	250–500 mg qid × 7 d
	2 g + 1 g probenecid	
Trimethoprim/Sulfamethoxazole	320/1600	320/1600 bid × 3 d

Data from Patterson TF, Andriole VT. Detection, significance, and therapy of bacteriuria in pregnancy. Update in the managed health care era. Infect Disclin North Am 1997;11(3):593–608; Le J, Briggs GG, Mckeown A, et al. Urinary tract infections during pregnancy. Ann Pharmacother 2004;38(10):1692–701; Connolly A, Thorp JM Jr. Urinary tract infections in pregnancy. Urol Clin North Am 1999;26(4):779–87; Ovalle A, Levancini M. Urinary tract infections in pregnancy. Curr Opin Urol 2001;11(1):55–9.

Upper UTI (acute pyelonephritis)

Epidemiology

Incidence of pyelonephritis during pregnancy is approximately 1% to 2%. However, 20% to 40% of women with untreated bacteriuria will develop pyelonephritis during pregnancy [1]. Pyelonephritis is seen most commonly during the third trimester, when stasis and hydronephrosis are most evident [3].

Diagnosis

Bacteriuria and clinical signs and symptoms establish a diagnosis of pyelonephritis. The signs and symptoms are similar to those of nonpregnant women, and include fever, nausea, vomiting, chills, and costovertebral tenderness.

Significance

In the preantimicrobial era, between 20% to 50% of children born to women with pyelonephritis were premature [42]. It has been theorized that the mechanism of preterm labor is associated with microorganism production of phospholipase A2 and subsequent prostaglandin activation [26]. Other reported complications of pyelonephritis have included low birth weight and neonatal death [42]. Although the complications of untreated pyelonephritis in pregnancy are well-known, there is debate in the literature as to whether antibiotic-treated pyelonephritis leads to adverse pregnancy outcomes.

Multiple maternal complications of pyelonephritis have also been reported, including anemia, hypertension [42], transient renal failure, acute respiratory distress syndrome, and sepsis [1].

Treatment

All patients who have pyelonephritis during pregnancy should be admitted and treated with parenteral agents [3]. Initial antimicrobial therapy is typically ampicillin plus gentamicin or cephalosporins. Second- or third-generation cephalosporins may also be considered for single-agent therapy [1]. With these treatment regimens, more than 95% of women will respond within 72 hours [43,44]. Resistant organisms must be considered in women who do not respond appropriately to treatment, and antimicrobials should be changed according to culture results. If treatment response is suboptimal despite culture-specific treatment, an ultrasound should be obtained to rule out nephrolithiasis, structural abnormality, or renal abscess [45].

Once afebrile, women may be switched to a 2-week outpatient course of an oral antimicrobial. This course should be followed by suppressive therapy until delivery [46,47]. As with ASB and cystitis, follow-up after treatment is important. Women should be monitored closely throughout their pregnancy because there is an increased risk of recurrent pyelonephritis [42].

Summary

UTIs are common complications of pregnancy and may lead to significant morbidity for both mother and fetus. During pregnancy, ASB is the major risk factor for developing a symptomatic UTI. Screening and treatment of pregnant women for ASB may prevent morbidity associated with symptomatic UTIs. Bacteriuria should be treated with short-course therapy with appropriate anti-microbials. Women should be followed closely after treatment of bacteriuria because recurrence may occur in up to one third of patients.

Key points in this article may be summarized as follows:

- Urine culture is the gold standard for screening for bacteriuria in pregnancy.
- All pregnant women should be screened for bacteriuria in the first trimester.
- Women with a history of recurrent UTI or urinary tract anomalies should have repeat bacteriuria screening throughout pregnancy.
- All bacteriuria should be treated during pregnancy.
- Treatment should be effective, and nontoxic to the fetus.
- Antimicrobial prophylaxis or close follow-up after treatment of ASB and symptomatic UTI is necessary throughout the remainder of pregnancy.

References

[1] Gilstrap LC 3rd, Ramin SM. Urinary tract infections during pregnancy. Obstet Gynecol Clin North Am 2001;28(3):581–91.

[2] Patterson TF, Andriole VT. Detection, significance, and therapy of bacteriuria in pregnancy. Update in the managed health care era. Infect Dis Clin North Am 1997;11(3):593–608.

[3] Schaeffer AJ. Infections of the urinary tract. In: Walsh PC, Retik AB, Vaughan ED Jr, et al, editors. Campbell's Urology. 8th edition. Philadelphia: WB Saunders; 2002. p. 516–602.

[4] Millar LK, Cox SM. Urinary tract infections complicating pregnancy. Infect Dis Clin North Am 1997;11(1):13–26.

[5] Gilbert GL, Garland SM, Fairley KF, et al. Bacteriuria due to ureaplasmas and other fastidious organisms during pregnancy: prevalence and significance. Pediatr Infect Dis 1986;5(6 Suppl):S239–43.

[6] Cohen I, Veille JC, Calkins BM. Improved pregnancy outcome following successful treatment of chlamydial infection. JAMA 1990;263(23):3160–3.

[7] Sweet RL. Bacteriuria and pyelonephritis during pregnancy. Semin Perinatol 1977;1(1):25–40.

[8] Krieger JN. Complications and treatment of urinary tract infections during pregnancy. Urol Clin North Am 1986;13(4):685–93.

[9] Waltzer WC. The urinary tract in pregnancy. J Urol 1981;125(3):271–6.

[10] Christensen B. Which antibiotics are appropriate for treating bacteriuria in pregnancy? J Antimicrob Chemother 2000;46(Suppl 1):29–34 [discussion 63–5].

[11] Dashe JS, Gilstrap LC 3rd. Antibiotic use in pregnancy. Obstet Gynecol Clin North Am 1997;24(3):617–29.

[12] Philipson A. Pharmacokinetics of ampicillin during pregnancy. J Infect Dis 1977;136(3):370–6.

[13] Stratton CW, Quinn J, Peterson L. Emerging resistance in uropathogens: its impact on management of acute cystitis in women [special issue]. Postgrad Med S 1994;31:1–23.

[14] Hooton TM, Stamm WE. Diagnosis and treatment of uncomplicated urinary tract infection. Infect Dis Clin North Am 1997;11(3):551–81.

[15] McFadyen IR, Campbell-Brown M, Stephenson M, et al. Single-dose treatment of bacteriuria in pregnancy. Eur Urol 1987;13(Suppl 1):22–5.

[16] Dinsmoor MJ, Gibbs RS. The role of the newer antimicrobial agents in obstetrics and gynecology. Clin Obstet Gynecol 1988;31(2):423–34.

[17] Reeves DS. A perspective on the safety of antibacterials used to treat urinary tract infections. J Antimicrob Chemother 1994;33(Suppl A):111–20.

[18] Keenan C. Prevention of neonatal group B streptococcal infection. Am Fam Physician 1998;57(11):2713–20.

[19] Weiser ACSA. The use and misuse of antimicrobial agents in urology. AUA Update Series 2002;31:137.

[20] MacLean AB. Urinary tract infection in pregnancy. Int J Antimicrob Agents 2001;17(4):273–6 [discussion 6–7].

[21] Porter PJ, Sweeney EA, Golan H, et al. Controlled study of the effect of prenatal tetracycline on primary dentition. Antimicrobial Agents Chemother (Bethesda) 1965;5:668–71.

[22] Whalley PJ, Adams RH, Combes B. Tetracycline toxicity in pregnancy. Liver and pancreatic dysfunction. JAMA 1964;189:357–62.

[23] Rubin RH, Shapiro ED, Andriole VT, et al. Evaluation of new anti-infective drugs for the treatment of urinary tract infection. Infectious Diseases Society of America and the Food and Drug Administration. Clin Infect Dis 1992;15(Suppl 1):S216–27.

[24] Stamey T. Pathogenesis and treatment of urinary tract infections. Baltimore: Williams & Wilkins; 1980.

[25] Turck M, Goffe BS, Petersdorf RG. Bacteriuria of pregnancy. Relation to socioeconomic factors. N Engl J Med 1962;266:857–60.

[26] Lucas MJ, Cunningham FG. Urinary infection in pregnancy. Clin Obstet Gynecol 1993;36(4):855–68.

[27] Kass EH. Bacteriuria and pyelonephritis of pregnancy. Arch Intern Med 1960;105:194–8.

[28] Harris RE. The significance of eradication of bacteriuria during pregnancy. Obstet Gynecol 1979;53(1):71–3.

[29] Schieve LA, Handler A, Hershow R, et al. Urinary tract infection during pregnancy: its association with maternal morbidity and perinatal outcome. Am J Public Health 1994;84(3):405–10.

[30] Stenqvist K, Dahlen-Nilsson I, Lidin-Janson G, et al. Bacteriuria in pregnancy. Frequency and risk of acquisition. Am J Epidemiol 1989;129(2):372–9.

[31] Kass E. Horatio at the orifice: the significance of bacteriuria. J Infec Dis 1978;138:546.

[32] Nicolle LE. Asymptomatic bacteriuria: when to screen and when to treat. Infect Dis Clin North Am 2003;17(2):367–94.

[33] Gratacos E, Torres PJ, Vila J, et al. Screening and treatment of asymptomatic bacteriuria in pregnancy prevent pyelonephritis. J Infect Dis 1994;169(6): 1390–2.

[34] Norden CW, Kass EH. Bacteriuria of pregnancy– a critical appraisal. Annu Rev Med 1968;19:431–70.

[35] McNair RD, MacDonald SR, Dooley SL, et al. Evaluation of the centrifuged and Gram-stained smear, urinalysis, and reagent strip testing to detect asymptomatic bacteriuria in obstetric patients. Am J Obstet Gynecol 2000;182(5):1076–9.

[36] Wadland WC, Plante DA. Screening for asymptomatic bacteriuria in pregnancy. A decision and cost analysis. J Fam Pract 1989;29(4):372–6.

[37] Campbell-Brown M, McFadyen IR. Bacteriuria in pregnancy treated with a single dose of cephalexin. Br J Obstet Gynaecol 1983;90(11):1054–9.

[38] Stamm WE, Hooton TM. Management of urinary tract infections in adults. N Engl J Med 1993; 329(18):1328–34.

[39] Andriole VT. Urinary tract infections in pregnancy. Urol Clin North Am 1975;2(3):485–98.

[40] Pfau A, Sacks TG. Effective prophylaxis for recurrent urinary tract infections during pregnancy. Clin Infect Dis 1992;14(4):810–4.

[41] Diokno AC, Compton A, Seski J, et al. Urologic evaluation of urinary tract infection in pregnancy. J Reprod Med 1986;31(1):23–6.

[42] Gilstrap LC, Leveno KJ, Cunningham FG, et al. Renal infection and pregnancy outcome. Am J Obstet Gynecol 1981;141(6):709–16.

[43] Cunningham FG, Morris GB, Mickal A. Acute pyelonephritis of pregnancy: a clinical review. Obstet Gynecol 1973;42(1):112–7.

[44] Sanchez-Ramos L, McAlpine KJ, Adair CD, et al. Pyelonephritis in pregnancy: once-a-day ceftriaxone versus multiple doses of cefazolin. A randomized, double-blind trial. Am J Obstet Gynecol 1995; 172(1 Pt 1):129–33.

[45] Connolly A, Thorp JM Jr. Urinary tract infections in pregnancy. Urol Clin North Am 1999;26(4):779–87.

[46] Faro S, Pastorek JG 2nd, Plauche WC, et al. Short-course parenteral antibiotic therapy for pyelonephritis in pregnancy. South Med J 1984;77(4): 455–7.

[47] Sandberg T, Brorson JE. Efficacy of long-term antimicrobial prophylaxis after acute pyelonephritis in pregnancy. Scand J Infect Dis 1991;23(2):221–3.

ELSEVIER
SAUNDERS

Urol Clin N Am 34 (2007) 43–52

UROLOGIC
CLINICS
of North America

Urolithiasis in Pregnancy

Vernon M. Pais, Jr, MD*, Alice L. Payton, MD,
Chad A. LaGrange, MD

Division of Urology, Department of Surgery, University of Kentucky College of Medicine,
University of Kentucky Chandler Medical Center, 800 Rose Street, Room MS-277, Lexington, KY 40536, USA

Epidemiology

The reported incidence of urolithiasis in pregnancy varies widely from 1 in 200 to 1 in 2000 pregnancies, although 1/1500 is frequently cited [1,2]. Overall, it is unlikely that pregnancy increases the incidence of stone disease despite several physiologic changes that theoretically could increase the risk for stone formation. When compared with nonpregnant age-matched controls, pregnant women do not have an elevated incidence of urolithiasis [3,4]. The true incidence is difficult to study, however, because typically only symptomatic stones are diagnosed in pregnant women, whereas in the general population stone disease is also diagnosed as an incidental finding on imaging studies. Stones in pregnancy may become symptomatic more frequently because of the physiologic dilatation of the collecting systems allowing for migration of renal stones into the ureter, leading to obstruction and pain [5]. Twice as many stones are found in the ureter as in the kidney at diagnosis, although this may simply represent the selective diagnosis of only those stones causing symptoms or obstruction during pregnancy.

As seen in the general population, the incidence of stone disease in pregnancy is higher in the southern United States and mountainous regions, and may be more frequent in white and Hispanic populations [6]. Symptomatic stone disease presents in the second or third trimester in 80% to 90% of women. Women who have

known recurrent stone disease do not appear to have an increased rate of stone formation during pregnancy [7].

Stones affect the two kidneys with equal frequency, even though physiologic hydronephrosis of pregnancy more commonly affects the right side [3]. No major differences in stone composition have been found when comparing pregnant women to the general population [8]. Most are calcium stones. Only 5% to 10% of these are believed to be secondary to hyperparathyroidism. The incidence of struvite stones is also similar to that in nonpregnant women. As with the general population, pregnant women who have struvite stones often present with urinary tract infection rather than renal colic [9].

Anatomic changes in the urinary tract

Significant anatomic and functional changes occur in the urinary tract during pregnancy. Of these, hydronephrosis has particular relevance in the diagnosis and presentation of urolithiasis. Hydronephrosis occurs in up to 90% of right kidneys and 67% of left kidneys in pregnant women [10]. Upper tract dilatation is usually present by 6 to 10 weeks' gestation and may persist until up to 6 weeks after delivery. Some studies show an increased incidence of hydronephrosis in nulliparous women, which may be secondary to stronger abdominal musculature that is less accommodating to an enlarging uterus [11]. Although physiologic hydronephrosis of pregnancy is typically asymptomatic, it may uncommonly present with renal colic [12]. Regardless, unilateral flank pain associated with hydronephrosis should raise one's suspicion of ureteral stone.

---

* Corresponding author.
E-mail address: vmpais2@email.uky.edu (V.M. Pais).

Both anatomic and physiologic causes for hydronephrosis of pregnancy have been proposed. One likely factor is extrinsic obstruction of the ureter by the gravid uterus against the fixed pelvic brim. The left ureter may be more protected from this compression by the left colon, accounting for the higher incidence on the right side. Also, the right ureter may be more frequently compressed by the engorged right uterine vein [3]. Ureteral dilatation is generally not present below the level of the uterus at the pelvic brim. Some have attributed this to restriction by Waldeyer's sheath around the distal ureter [13]. Ureters that do not cross the pelvic brim, such as those associated with ectopic and pelvic kidneys and nonorthotopic urinary diversions, typically do not have significant dilation in pregnancy, lending further support to a mechanical cause [8,9]. Hormones, especially progesterone, may also contribute to hydronephrosis of pregnancy. Progesterone decreases ureteral peristalsis and relaxes the ureteral smooth muscle. Evidence supporting a hormonal influence includes the finding that some women have ureteral dilatation seen by ultrasound during the first trimester, before the uterus has reached the level of the pelvic brim to cause mechanical obstruction [11]. Other evidence for hormonal influence is the development of hydronephrosis in pregnant rats. Because the uterus hangs anteriorly in quadrupeds, it is not expected to cause obstruction. Also, the rats' renal pelvic pressure studies confirmed nonobstructive dilatation [14].

Physiologic changes during pregnancy

Of the various physiologic changes of pregnancy, some significantly alter the risk for stone formation. Others have no direct effect on urolithiasis, but are important for planning surgical intervention and pre- and postoperative care in pregnant women. These changes are reviewed elsewhere in this volume, so only a brief overview follows.

Pregnancy is a hypercoagulable state with increased risk for deep venous thrombosis and embolism. Several factors contribute to this increased risk, including increased production of clotting factors and fibrinogen, decreased fibrinolytic activity, and possibly compression of the inferior vena cava by the gravid uterus causing venous stasis.

The effects to the respiratory system increase the anesthetic risk. The functional reserve capacity of the lungs is decreased in the gravid state, yet the consumption of oxygen is increased. Hypoxemia is thus a risk if not appropriately ventilated.

Pregnancy also confers an increased risk for aspiration during general anesthesia. The gravid uterus causes increased intra-abdominal pressure, whereas progesterone decreases gastric emptying and causes relaxation of the lower esophageal sphincter.

The cardiovascular system must change to accommodate the developing fetus. The heart becomes hyperdynamic to meet the increased metabolic demand of pregnancy with a 30% to 50% increase in cardiac output. Total blood volume is also increased by 25% to 40%, with plasma volume increased disproportionately to red blood cell mass leading to hemodilution and physiologic anemia of pregnancy [15].

Pregnancy induces significant changes in renal physiology. Increased cardiac output leads to increased renal plasma flow and glomerular filtration rate (GFR), which usually peaks at 9 to 11 weeks' gestation and resolves postpartum [1]. Total urine volume is essentially unchanged [6]. The increased GFR leads to a 25% decrease in normal values for serum creatinine and blood urea nitrogen, so a serum creatinine of greater than 0.8 in a pregnant woman may be considered elevated. Also, dose adjustments in consultation with the obstetrician and pharmacist may be needed for medications that are eliminated by glomerular filtration because of increased renal clearance of these drugs.

Pathophysiology of urolithiasis in pregnancy

Myriad metabolic conditions affect the risk for urolithiasis. Of these, the three that occur most often in pregnancy are hypercalciuria, hyperuricosuria, and hypercitraturia.

Hypercalciuria

The cause of hypercalciuria of pregnancy is multifactorial. GFR increases in pregnancy. The subsequent increase in tubular flow leads to decreased tubular reabsorption and increased net excretion of calcium. Also, placental formation of 1,25-dihydroxycholecalciferol promotes intestinal reabsorption of calcium and mobilization of calcium from bone [16]. Feedback mechanisms suppress the production of parathyroid hormone. This suppression may cause a two- to threefold decrease in the tubular reabsorption of calcium, contributing further to hypercalciuria [12]. Despite the increased urine calcium excretion, the serum calcium levels remain near normal because of the balance between increased intestinal absorption and increased renal loss, essentially mimicking absorptive hypercalciuria. Additionally, some pregnant women use high-calcium diets and supplements [16,17].

Hyperuricosuria

Hyperuricosuria may also occur during pregnancy [7,12]. It has been attributed to the increased GFR and subsequent increase in net urinary excretion of uric acid. Even in those who do not have uric acid urolithiasis, hyperuricosuria is of clinical importance because it is a well-recognized risk factor for calcium oxalate nephrolithiasis [18]. Hyperuricosuria has been previously implicated as a contributory factor in calcium urolithiasis and the accelerated stent encrustation of pregnancy [12].

Hypercitraturia

Citrate prevents urolithiasis by way of multiple mechanisms. Complexed with calcium, it is more soluble than other calcium salts. Additionally, citrate can act as an inhibitor of crystal growth and aggregation. Citrate depletion is a known cause of urolithiasis in the general population; however, in pregnancy urine citrate is increased [6,12]. The increased urinary citrate likely has a clinically significant protective effect, offsetting the effects of hypercalciuria and hyperuricosuria. Although citrate is one of the most well-recognized inhibitors of stone formation, others, including magnesium and glycoproteins, may also serve a protective role during pregnancy [8].

Complex changes occur during pregnancy, which may affect the risk for stone formation. Homogeneous crystal nucleation may result from urinary supersaturation of the involved crystal, accentuated by the previously noted hypercalciuria and hyperuricosuria. Also, uric acid crystals may allow heterogeneous nucleation and epitaxial crystal growth of calcium oxalate. It has been suggested that the hydronephrosis of pregnancy may allow sufficient stasis of urine to facilitate crystal retention and further growth [9]. Nevertheless it is generally accepted that pregnancy is not a state of increased stone formation. Even patients who have a known history of stone disease do not show increased rates of urolithiasis during pregnancy [7]. The precise reasons that pregnancy is

not a state of accelerated stone formation are not fully understood, but likely relate to increased inhibitory activity and the limited duration of pregnancy.

Clinical presentation of stone disease in pregnancy

In many cases the classic presentation of renal colic because of an obstructing calculus is unmistakable. Symptomatic urolithiasis in the expectant mother may present differently than in the nonpregnant patient, however. Additionally, pregnant women may suffer from abdominal and flank pain, nausea, emesis, and irritative lower urinary tract symptoms unrelated to urolithiasis. The anatomic changes that occur in the gravid abdomen and pelvis can alter the perception, radiation, and localization of pain, making the clinical assessment of abdominal pain difficult [9]. Prompt diagnosis is important, as delay could potentially have untoward effects on kidney function and maternal and fetal health [19]. It is thus imperative that the practitioner consider stone disease in pregnant women who have abdominal or flank discomfort or lower urinary tract symptoms.

In general, patients present with stone symptoms in the second or third trimesters of pregnancy. At this point in pregnancy, the gravid uterus has enlarged above the pelvic brim and may be impinging on the distal ureter. The most common symptoms of renal or ureteral stones in pregnancy are flank or abdominal pain, microscopic or gross hematuria, and irritative lower urinary tract symptoms. Presenting symptoms may vary depending on the clinical scenario. For example, ureteral stones are more likely to present with classic renal colic. Distal stones may elicit more irritative voiding symptoms [5]. Struvite stones may present with urinary tract infection rather than renal colic [9]. Hydronephrosis of pregnancy may occasionally present with abdominal or flank pain, mimicking stone disease [20,21]. Other kidney conditions, such as renal vein thrombosis or acute pyelonephritis, may also cause flank or abdominal pain [22]. Pain caused by appendicitis, cholecystitis, diverticulitis, and placental disorders may present with pain in nontypical areas of the abdomen or flank because of displacement of these organs by the gravid uterus [15].

Signs of urolithiasis include hematuria, pyuria, or obstetric complications. Hematuria may signify stone disease and other conditions associated with pregnancy. Physiologic hydronephrosis of pregnancy can cause rupture of small veins in the renal pelvis or pyramids leading to hematuria [9]. Urinary tract infections are also frequently associated with hematuria, especially if the patient has a history of congenital or acquired urinary tract anomalies. Other possible causes of hematuria in pregnancy include renovascular complications, renal tumor, urothelial tumor, and endometriosis [13]. Up to 42% of pregnant women who have renal colic and urolithiasis have pyuria at presentation [23]. Patients who have urinary tract infections who remain febrile for more than 48 hours should be further evaluated for complicated urinary tract infections attributable to urolithiasis [9]. With regard to obstetric complications, renal colic may induce premature onset of labor, which may be stopped by pain control or spontaneous stone passage [9]. Women who have obstructive uropathy may also present with preeclampsia or isolated hypertension. This hypertension has been successfully alleviated with relief of the obstruction [24].

Diagnostic imaging

Radiographic imaging is important for treatment planning and diagnosis. Therapy can be planned based on estimation of renal function, stone size, location, configuration, and potential composition—all information gleaned from appropriately selected radiographic studies. Conversely, some of these studies have limited or no use in pregnant women because of concerns regarding fetal risk.

When clinical circumstances require imaging, an understanding of the inherent risks and benefits may help alleviate the anxiety of the patient and the physician. The effects of cumulative and threshold doses on fetal risk, the gestational age at which these risks are most pronounced, and the dose delivered by the respective studies are all considered. Some studies can be tailored to reduce fetal risk. Taking all of this into account, one may formulate a plan for using these studies in properly selected patients.

Radiation-induced risks

Cell death and teratogenic effects are believed to have a threshold dose below which these effects are unlikely to occur, but above which there may be increasing severity with increasing exposure. Such effects include intrauterine growth retardation and mental retardation. High doses of radiation before implantation and during the first 2 weeks postconception are most likely to result in fetal loss [9]. During the 4- to 10-week gestational period of organogenesis the fetus is most susceptible to the teratogenic effects of radiation. Doses of less than 5 cGy are not believed to cause intrauterine growth retardation or other fetal anomalies [3,25]. This dose thus represents what is generally considered to be the maximum safe dose, below which there is no specific association of fetal anomalies or pregnancy loss [25]. Mental retardation has a proposed threshold dose of 20 cGy. The risk for such central nervous system damage seems to be greatest between 8 and 15 weeks' gestational age, as determined by studies of atomic bomb survivors [3,25]. The risk for severe mental retardation climbs with increasing dose, reaching 40% and 60% at doses of 100 and 150 cGy, respectively [25].

The risks of cancer and genetic mutations may also increase with increasing radiation dose, although this is still debated. Fetal exposure to 1 to 2 cGy has been believed to increase the rate of childhood leukemia from the background rate of 1 in 3000 to 1 in 2000 [25]. A critical review of the original studies noted flawed methodology and failed to identify a solid basis for concerns regarding the induction of leukemia [26]. An estimated 50 to 100 cGy, far in excess of the doses encountered in diagnostic studies, is required to double the baseline genetic mutation rate [3].

The delivered dose of radiation varies with the study performed. Most uroradiologic studies can be modified to be performed within the aforementioned 5-cGy limit. This limit can be surpassed, however, with standard computed tomography or excessive fluoroscopy; thus communication with the radiologist is suggested. Also, the actual radiation dose delivered to the fetus is affected by the mother's body size and the depth of the fetus from her skin at the site of radiation entrance. Consultation with a radiation physicist is therefore helpful to calculate the estimated delivered dose.

Use of radiographic studies

Ultrasound

For most pregnant women who have possible urolithiasis, evaluation may proceed without radiation exposure. Ultrasound shows the renal parenchyma, calyces, and pelvis. Significant renal cortical thinning may suggest chronic obstruction.

Dilation of the calyces and renal pelvis is also easily seen. Falsely positive and negative interpretation of hydronephrosis may occur, however. Nonobstructive caliectasis and parapelvic cysts may be mistaken for obstructive hydronephrosis. Conversely, if ultrasound is performed too early in the course of obstruction or in the setting of dehydration, significant dilation may not be visualized. This problem is underscored by a reported false negative rate of 35% in the setting of acute obstruction with conventional ultrasound [27]. In pregnant patients, the high prevalence of physiologic hydronephrosis further complicates the interpretation. In hydronephrosis of pregnancy, however, ureteral dilation is only above the pelvic brim. If the ureteral dilation extends below the pelvic brim one should consider distal ureteral obstruction.

Currently the most promising modification of ultrasonography to better discern obstruction is Doppler ultrasonography, which adds a functional element to the evaluation of the kidney. With Doppler techniques the velocity of intrarenal blood flow can be quantitated and the resistive index (RI) can be calculated. The RI is defined as the peak systolic velocity (PSV) minus the end-diastolic velocity (EDV), divided by the peak systolic velocity: $(PSV - EDV)/PSV$.

In the general population, the role of RI in assessing for obstruction is controversial [28–30]. RI may have a special usefulness in the pregnant population, however. RI does not appear to be affected by nonobstructive hydronephrosis of pregnancy [31,32]. In one study, the difference in RI between the affected and unaffected kidney was highly accurate in identifying ureteral obstruction attributable to stone disease in pregnant women. Women who had obstruction had a difference in RI of 0.06, compared with 0.006 in women who did not have obstruction [32]. Although larger studies are clearly needed, Doppler ultrasonography holds significant promise in the evaluation of urolithiasis and in the differentiation of stone obstruction from hydronephrosis of pregnancy.

Excretory urography

The excretory urogram (EXU) or intravenous pyelogram provides anatomic evaluation of radiopaque structures and may reveal radiolucent structures within the urinary tract as filling defects. EXU also provides a functional assessment of the kidney. Its reliance on glomerular filtration and renal excretion of the contrast agent limits its use in those who have renal insufficiency or contrast allergy. The standard EXU, which typically incorporates scout films, tomograms, and multiple timed images, must be tailored to minimize radiation exposure to the fetus. A proposed protocol includes a scout film followed by a 30-minute film. If insufficient information can be gleaned from these, the acquisition of additional films should be based on the 30-minute film. A faint nephrogram suggesting a high-grade obstruction may prompt a 2- to 3-hour delayed film. Conversely, a dense nephrogram may prompt an earlier, 1-hour follow-up film [2]. Additional measures include judicious collimation, short exposure times, maximal fetal shielding, and prone positioning [9]. With such measures, the exposure may be potentially limited to approximately 1 to 2 cGy.

The iodinated contrast used for EXU has been shown to cross the placenta. Although mutagenic and teratogenic effects have not been demonstrated, free iodide may potentially depress fetal thyroid function. It has thus been recommended by the Contrast Media Safety Committee of the European Society of Urogenital Radiology to check neonatal thyroid function during the first week postpartum [33].

CT

In 1995, Smith and colleagues demonstrated the superior accuracy of CT compared with routine EXU in diagnosing ureteral calculi [34]. Because of its increased speed, elimination of intravenous contrast, and superior sensitivity, the unenhanced helical CT has become the gold standard for diagnosis of a suspected ureteral stone. This paradigm shift in imaging has not extended to pregnant women, however, because the estimated radiation dose to the fetus approaches 3.5 cGy on conventional scanners [25]. Renal stone protocol CT on newer multidetector scanners has potential radiation doses of 0.88 to 1.2 cGy [35]. Low-dose and ultra–low-dose CT protocols have been developed to further limit delivered radiation dose. Recently presented but unpublished data reported 15 women undergoing low-dose stone protocol CT during pregnancy, receiving a mean exposure of 0.721 cGy [36]. At present, such techniques remain second-line diagnostic studies, reserved only for those in whom an adequate treatment plan cannot be determined based on clinical examination and ultrasonography. With further evolution of techniques and continued diminishment of dose, CT may become more widely used in this population.

MRI

MRI provides detailed, cross-sectional images without exposure to ionizing radiation. As such, it has been advocated as a nonradiating, noninvasive way to investigate ureteral obstruction in pregnant women. Typically, hydronephrosis of pregnancy is seen as hydroureter to the level of the pelvic brim, probably by compressing the ureter between the pelvic brim and the uterus [21]. Conversely, a "double kink sign," noted by a standing column of urine to the pelvic brim and a second column of urine from the brim to the presumed distal ureteral obstruction, suggests a distal ureteral stone [21]. In a nonpregnant population, diuretic MRU had 93% accuracy for obstruction attributable to stone, whereas EXU had 96% accuracy [37].

Unfortunately, calculi do not have a distinct appearance on MRI, as they do on CT. Instead, obstruction by stone, clot, or other intraureteral lesion must be inferred from the presence of a ureteral filling defect on high-resolution T2 images. Although protocols have been demonstrated to accurately depict the presence and level of ureteral obstruction, the specific cause of obstruction may remain elusive. Other limitations of MRI include the time and cost incurred in acquisition of these images. Nevertheless, MRI continues to emerge as a useful adjunctive study in the evaluation of pregnant women who have abdominal pain. Additionally, it potentially allows the diagnosis of other clinically important causes of pain including ovarian torsion and appendicitis [38].

Currently, ultrasound remains an appropriate first-line imaging study in the pregnant patient who has possible urolithiasis. When second-line studies are necessary, several options are available. A limited excretory urogram, MR urogram, or the emerging ultra–low-dose tailored CT may be considered in these cases. The selection of the best second-line study will depend on the local institution's capabilities and should be performed in consultation with the obstetrician and radiologist.

Management of urolithiasis in pregnancy

The management of a symptomatic stone diagnosed during pregnancy poses multiple challenges to the patient, obstetrician, and urologist. An understanding of the natural history of urolithiasis in pregnancy and the limitations imposed by the pregnancy aids in the formulation of a rational approach to each patient.

Expectant management

Most stones will pass spontaneously, as supported by several of the larger studies, published to date. Parulkar and colleagues [39] reported 64% of their 70 patients passed their stones without surgical intervention. Others with series of 80 to 90 patients were even more encouraging: 70% to 84% passed their stones with expectant management [23,40]. For stones that do not pass during pregnancy, about 50% will pass in the postpartum period [23]. It is our practice to obtain a stone protocol CT scan in the postpartum period for those who did not definitively pass the stone before delivery.

Expectant management includes appropriate hydration and analgesia. Urine should be strained so that stone passage may be documented. Antibiotics are given for those with documented bacteriuria or findings suggestive of a potential urinary tract infection [19]. Expectant therapy, although nonoperative, may be nevertheless active. Approximately one third of patients managed in this fashion require multiple admissions, many of which may be prolonged given the need for fetal monitoring and extended periods of intravenous hydration [40]. As this may be expected for a significant minority of patients, repeated admissions alone should not be considered an absolute criterion for surgical intervention.

This conservative policy of watchful waiting with supportive care, in either an inpatient or outpatient setting as necessary, is espoused as initial management for all except those who have clinical indications to intervene.

Expulsive therapy

The use of oral calcium channel blockers, alpha blockers, and corticosteroids to facilitate stone passage has increased significantly in recent years. The first two measures mechanistically aim to diminish distal ureteral smooth muscle tone and spasm, whereas the steroids may reduce edema of the distal ureter. In nonpregnant patients, placebo controlled trials showed significantly increased rates of stone passage and decreased time until stone passage [41,42]. To date, however, neither efficacy nor safety in the pregnant population has been demonstrated.

An epidural block has been suggested as an alternate way to reduce distal ureteral smooth muscle tone. In addition to providing excellent pain relief, it may reduce ureteral spasm and facilitate stone passage. In two series of non-pregnant patients, the majority passed their stones after epidural block, unless the stone was known to be impacted [43,44]. Epidural blocks are commonly used to reduce the pain of childbearing and their safety for mother and fetus are well accepted, provided that maternal hypotension is avoided [45]. There is only one report of using epidural anesthesia to facilitate stone passage in a pregnant woman. The block was maintained for 18 hours, with full resolution of pain and emesis. A healthy term infant was born. Definitive passage of the stone was not confirmed, only presumed because of full resolution of symptoms [46]. Although infrequently used, this may be of benefit for select patients who fail more conservative expectant management when operative intervention is not possible because of patient refusal or the lack of equipment or endourologic expertise.

Surgical management

Despite attempts at conservative management, surgical intervention may ultimately be required. Absolute indications to intervene parallel those in the nonpregnant patient, and include febrile urinary tract infection, pyonephrosis, or sepsis, obstruction of a solitary kidney, intractable pain, nausea, or vomiting. Selection of the appropriate intervention must take into consideration the capabilities and limitations of the institution and should respect the wishes of the patient and comfort level and clinical judgment of the urologist, obstetrician, and anesthesiologist.

Indwelling ureteral stent placement

Retrograde placement of an indwelling ureteral stent for obstruction during pregnancy is well established [47]. It is a procedure routinely performed by most urologists and the equipment is readily available at most centers. Its efficacy in relieving obstruction is well recognized [4]. Additionally, ureteral stent placement can be potentially performed under local anesthesia with ultrasonic rather than fluoroscopic guidance [4].

Limitations of stent placement in pregnancy are also well known. Although most urologists are adept at fluoroscopic stent placement, ultrasound-guided positioning may be unfamiliar to many, thus necessitating limited fluoroscopy or the assistance of an ultrasound technician and radiologist. Irritative lower urinary tract symptoms

attributable to the stent are common. Also, rapid stent encrustation is often observed and has been attributed to hypercalciuria and hyperuricosuria of pregnancy [12,48]. To avoid stent encrustation, some urologists recommend stent exchange every 4 to 8 weeks [8]. For this reason, some algorithms have advocated nephrostomy tube placement in early pregnancy (before 22 weeks' gestation) and ureteral stents thereafter so as to avoid the need for an excessive number of interventions over the course of the pregnancy [48].

Percutaneous nephrostomy

An alternative means of obtaining urinary drainage is the placement of a percutaneous nephrostomy tube. This procedure is routinely performed with local anesthesia under ultrasound guidance. At most centers, this requires the expertise of an interventional radiologist. Advantages include the ability to perform it even in the acutely ill under local anesthesia, avoidance of retrograde manipulation of the obstructed ureter and its associated potential for ureteral perforation, and the ability to immediately confirm and continually assess drainage of the obstructed system [49]. Obstruction is readily identifiable and may be managed by simple irrigation of the tube, followed by tube exchange over a guidewire if irrigation fails [50]. Finally, nephrostomy tube placement provides access for subsequent percutaneous nephrolithotomy in those patients whose stone burden mandates such therapy in the postpartum period [49].

As is the case with any foreign body in the urinary tract, encrustation may also occur on the nephrostomy tube. Disadvantages of external tubes are the inconvenience of dealing with a collection device, the risk for accidental dislodgement, and bacterial colonization. Kavoussi and colleagues [50] noted persistent, albeit asymptomatic, bacteriuria in each of their six pregnant patients who had nephrostomy tubes, despite the use of prophylactic antibiotics. Finally, percutaneous renal access may be complicated by significant bleeding because of tract creation and dilation.

Selection of urinary drainage

Prospective studies comparing ureteral stents with nephrostomy tubes have been conducted in nonpregnant patients. Overall, these studies found that internal ureteral stents had a statistically significant increase in irritative lower urinary tract symptoms compared with percutaneous nephrostomies [51]. Indwelling stents also were associated with increased analgesic requirements and decreased overall quality of life [52]. To date, however, comparison of these two modalities in pregnant women has not been performed in a prospective randomized trial.

If expectant management fails and urinary diversion is desired, the choice between nephrostomy tube and stent is made based on the aforementioned factors.

Ureteroscopy

With continued advancement in endoscopic technology and endourologic techniques, ureteroscopy has become less invasive and less traumatic, such that many now consider it a first-line treatment for pregnant patients who have failed expectant management [20,53]. Several small series have reported stone free rates ranging from 70% to 100%, with displacement of proximal ureteral stones into the kidney accounting for most residual calculi [20,53–55]. As described by Watterson and colleagues [53], ureteroscopy is performed under general anesthesia in a modified dorsal lithotomy position. The floppy tip guide or glidewire is passed into the ureteral orifice under direct vision, using fluoroscopy only if resistance to wire advancement is encountered. Either semirigid or flexible ureteroscopy can be performed, as dictated by the clinical circumstances. Stones amenable to basket extraction are removed intact. Currently, the holmium laser is the preferred means of lithotripsy for those stones that cannot be removed intact. The versatility of the holmium laser allows efficient lithotripsy of all stone compositions and its physics allow a large margin of safety, provided the tip is kept at least 1 mm from the ureteral wall [53]. In vitro studies suggest that the peak pressures generated by endoscopic lithotripsy are unlikely to damage fetal hearing, although the data are limited and largely theoretic [56]. The decision to proceed with endoscopic management of a ureteral stone during pregnancy should be determined by the clinical scenario, and the availability and expertise of urologic, obstetric, and anesthetic care.

Shock wave lithotripsy

Shock wave lithotripsy (SWL) requires a brief note. The mechanical effects of generated shock waves can have catastrophic effects on an intrauterine pregnancy. Animal studies have confirmed fetal death after exposure to SWL, although the effects appeared most prominent later in pregnancy [57]. A critical review of suggested contraindications confirmed that pregnancy remains a strict contraindication to SWL [58]. Occasionally, a patient who had undergone SWL may thereafter realize that she had an unrecognized pregnancy at the time of treatment. Case reports and small retrospective series have addressed this and have documented women who underwent SWL in their first trimester and subsequently delivered healthy infants without detectable malformation [59,60]. Although one certainly cannot advocate SWL during pregnancy, such reports should somewhat alleviate concerns if SWL occurs during an unrecognized pregnancy and should discourage routine termination of pregnancy otherwise based on a fear that a fetus would not survive SWL.

Summary

Urolithiasis in pregnancy remains a diagnostic and therapeutic challenge. Its presentation may mimic the normal findings of pregnancy and other retroperitoneal and intra-abdominal conditions. Ultrasonography remains the cornerstone of imaging; the role of MRI is continuing to evolve. Modifications of technique may allow safer use of EXU and ultra–low-dose CT as second-line studies when clinically indicated. As most stones will pass spontaneously, expectant management with supportive care should be attempted, but temporary urinary drainage and definitive ureteroscopic management are highly successful if required. Shock wave lithotripsy remains contraindicated in pregnancy. Although the expectant mother who has flank pain is often approached with trepidation, the combination of a high index of suspicion, careful regard for the mother and fetus, and use of well-established endourologic techniques maximizes the possibility of an excellent, stone free outcome.

References

[1] Gorton E, Whitfield H. Renal calculi in pregnancy. BJU 1997;80(Suppl 1):4–9.
[2] Drago JR, Rohner TJ, Chez RA. Management of urinary calculi in pregnancy. Urology 1982;20: 578–81.
[3] Biyani CS, Joyce AD. Urolithiasis in pregnancy I: pathophysiology, fetal considerations, and diagnosis. BJU Int 2002;89:811–8.
[4] Jarrard DJ, Gerber GS, Lyon ES. Management of acute ureteral obstruction in pregnancy utilizing ultrasound guided placement of ureteral stents. Urology 1993;42:263–7.

[5] Kroovand RL. Stones in pregnancy. In: Coe FL, Favus MJ, Pak CYC, Parks JH, Preminger GM, editors. Kidney stones: medical and surgical management. Philadelphia: Lippincott-Raven Publishers; 1996. p. 1059–64.

[6] Maikranz P, Coe F, Parks J, et al. Nephrolithiasis in pregnancy. Am J Kidney Dis 1987;9:354–8.

[7] Coe FL, Parks JA, Lindheimer MD. Nephrolithiasis during pregnancy. N Engl J Med 1978;298:324–6.

[8] McAleer S, Loughlin K. Nephrolithiasis and pregnancy. Curr Opin Urol 2004;14:123–7.

[9] Swanson SK, Heilman RL, Eversman WG. Urinary tract stones in pregnancy. Surg Clin North Am 1995; 75:123–42.

[10] Khoo L, Anson K, Patel U. Success and short-term complication rates of percutaneous nephrostomy during pregnancy. J Vasc Radiol 2004;15:1469–73.

[11] Faundes A, Bricola-Filho M, Pinto e Silva JL. Dilation of the urinary tract during pregnancy: proposal of a curve of maximal caliceal diameter by gestational age. Am J Obstet Gynecol 1998;178:1082–6.

[12] Goldfarb R, Neerhut G, Lederer E. Management of acute hydronephrosis of pregnancy by ureteral stenting: risk of stone formation. J Urol 1989;141:921–2.

[13] Waltzer W. The urinary tract in pregnancy. J Urol 1981;125:271–6.

[14] Hsia TY, Shortliffe LM. The effect of pregnancy on rat urinary tract dynamics. J Urol 1995;154:684–9.

[15] Loughlin K. Management of urologic problems during pregnancy. Urology 1994;44(2):159–69.

[16] Gertner JM, Coustan DR, Kliger AS, et al. Pregnancy as state of physiologic absorptive hypercalciuria. Am J Med 1986;81:451–6.

[17] Smith C, Kristensen C, Davis M, et al. An evaluation of the physicochemical risk for renal stone disease during pregnancy. Clin Nephrol 2001;55(3):205–11.

[18] Coe FL, Kavalich AG. Hypercalciuria and hyperuricosuria in patients with calcium nephrolithiasis. N Engl J Med 1974;291:1344–50.

[19] Hendricks SK, Ross SO, Krieger JN. An algorithm for diagnosis and therapy of management and complications of urolithiasis during pregnancy. Surg Gynecol Obstet 1991;172:49–54.

[20] Lifshitz DA, Lingeman JE. Ureteroscopy as a first line intervention for ureteral calculi in pregnancy. J Endourol 2002;16:19–22.

[21] Spencer JA, Chahal R, Kelly A, et al. Evaluation of painful hydronephrosis in pregnancy: magnetic resonance urographic patterns in physiological dilatation versus calculous obstruction. J Urol 2004;171: 256–60.

[22] Murthy L. Urinary tract obstruction during pregnancy: recent developments in imaging. BJU 1997; 80(Suppl 1):1–3.

[23] Stothers L, Lee LM. Renal colic in pregnancy. J Urol 1992;148:1383–7.

[24] Satin A, Seiken G, Cunningham F. Reversible hypertension in pregnancy caused by obstructive uropathy. Obstet Gynecol 1993;81:823–5.

[25] Bulletins ACOG. ACOG Committee Opinion No 299: Guidelines for diagnostic imaging during pregnancy. Obstet Gynecol 2004;104:647–51.

[26] Smits AK, Paladine HL, Judkins DZ. What are the risks to the fetus associated with diagnostic radiation exposure during pregnancy? J Fam Pract 2006;55: 441–4.

[27] Laing FC, Jeffrey RB, Wing VW. Ultrasound versus excretory urography in evaluating acute flank pain. Radiology 1985;154:613–6.

[28] Platt JF, Rubin JM, Ellis JH. Acute renal obstruction: evaluation with intrarenal duplex Doppler and conventional ultrasound. Radiology 1993;186:685–8.

[29] Tublin ME, Dodd GD, Verdile VP. Acute renal colic: diagnosis with duplex Doppler US. Radiology 1994;193:697–701.

[30] Chen JH, Pu YS, Liu SP, et al. Renal hemodynamics in patients with obstructive uropathy evaluated by duplex Doppler sonography. J Urol 1993;150:18–21.

[31] Nazarian GK, Platt JF, Rubin JM, et al. Renal duplex Doppler sonography in asymptomatic women during pregnancy. J Ultrasound Med 1993;12(8): 441–4.

[32] Shokeir AA, Mahran MR, Abdulmaaboud M. Renal colic in pregnant women: role of resistive index. Urology 2000;55(3):344–7.

[33] Webb JA, Thomsen HS, Morcos SK. The use of iodinated and gadolinium contrast media during pregnancy and lactation. Eur Radiol 2005;15:1234–40.

[34] Smith RC, Rosenfield AT, Choe KA, et al. Acute flank pain: comparison of non-contrast enhanced CT and intravenous urography. Radiology 1995; 194:789–94.

[35] Hurwitz LM, Yoshizumi T, Reiman RE, et al. Radiation dose to the fetus from body MDCT during early gestation. AJR 2006;186:871–6.

[36] White WM, Gash J, Hatcher P, et al. Low dose computerized tomography for the evaluation of flank pain in the pregnant population. Podium presentation 76, annual meeting of the SES AUA. Rio Grande, Puerto Rico; March 4, 2006.

[37] Karabacakoglu A, Karakose S, Ince O, et al. Diagnostic value of diuretic-enhanced excretory MR urography in patients with obstructive uropathy. Eur J Radiol 2004;52:320–7.

[38] Birchard KR, Brown MA, Hyslop WB, et al. MRI of acute abdominal and pelvic pain in pregnant patients. AJR 2005;184:452–8.

[39] Parulkar BG, Hopkins TB, Wollin MR, et al. Renal colic during pregnancy: a case for conservative treatment. J Urol 1998;159:365–8.

[40] Lewis DF, Robichaux AG, Jaekle RK, et al. Urolithiasis in pregnancy: diagnosis, management, and pregnancy outcome. J Reprod Med 2003;48:28–32.

[41] Dellabella M, Milanese G, Muzzonigro G. Efficacy of tamsulosin in the medical management of juxtavesical ureteral stones. J Urol 2003;170:2202–5.

[42] Dellabella M, Milanese G, Muzzonigro G. Medical-expulsive therapy for distal ureterolithiasis:

randomized prospective study on role of corticoste-roids used in combination with tamsulosin-simpli-fied treatment regimen and health-related quality of life. Urology 2005;66:712–5.

[43] Romagnoli A, Batra MS. Continuous epidural block in the treatment of impacted ureteric stones. Can Med Assoc J 1973;109:968.

[44] Olshwang D, Shapiro A, Perlberg S, et al. The effect of epidural morphine on ureteral colic and spasm of the bladder. Pain 1984;18:97–101.

[45] Scherer R, Holzgreve W. Influence of epidural anal-gesia on fetal and neonatal well-being. Eur J Obstet Gynecol Reprod Biol 1995;59(Suppl):S17–29.

[46] Ready LB, Johnson ES. Epidural block for treat-ment of renal colic during pregnancy. Canad. Anaesth. Soc. J 1981;28:77–9.

[47] Loughlin KR, Bailey RB. Internal ureteral stents for conservative management of ureteral calculi during pregnancy. N Engl J Med 1986;315:1647–9.

[48] Denstedt JD, Razvi H. Management of urinary cal-culi during pregnancy. J Urol 1992;148:1072–5.

[49] Biyani CS, Joyce AD. Urolithiasis in pregnancy II: management. BJU Int 2002;89:819–23.

[50] Kavoussi LR, Albala DM, Basler JW, et al. Percuta-neous management of urolithiasis during pregnancy. J Urol 1992;148:1069–71.

[51] Joshi HB, Adams S, Obadeyi OO, et al. Nephros-tomy tube or "JJ" ureteric stent in ureteric obstruc-tion: assessment of patient perspectives using quality of life survey and utility analysis. Eur Urol 2001;39: 695–701.

[52] Mokhmalji H, Braun PM, Portillo JM, et al. Percuta-neous nephrostomy versus ureteral stents for diversion of hydronephrosis caused by stones: a prospective, randomized clinical trial. J Urol 2001;165:1088–92.

[53] Watterson JD, Girvan AR, Beiko DT, et al. Ure-teroscopy and holmium: YAG laser lithotripsy: an emerging definitive management strategy for symp-tomatic ureteral calculi in pregnancy. Urology 2002;60:383–7.

[54] Carringer M, Swartz R, Johansson JE. Management of ureteric calculi in pregnancy by ureteroscopy and laser lithotripsy. Br J Urol 1996;77:17–20.

[55] Shokeir AA, Mutabagani H. Rigid ureteroscopy in pregnant women. Br J Urol 1998;81:678–81.

[56] Karlsen SJ, Bull-Njaa T, Krokstad A. Measurement of sound emission by endoscopic lithotripters: an in vitro study and theoretical estimation of risk of hear-ing loss in a fetus. J Endourol 2001;15:821–6.

[57] Yalcin O, Tahmaz L, Yumbul Z, et al. Effects of shock waves on the rat fetus. Scand J Urol Nephrol 1998;32:167–70.

[58] Streem S. Contemporary clinical practice of shock wave lithotripsy: a reevaluation of contraindica-tions. J Urol 1997;157:1197–203.

[59] Asgari MA, Safarinejad MR, Hosseini SY, et al. Ex-tracorporeal shock wave lithotripsy of renal calculi during early pregnancy. BJU Int 1999;84:615–7.

[60] Deliveliotis CH, Argyropoulos B, Chrisofos M, et al. Shockwave lithotripsy in unrecognized pregnancy: interruption or continuation? J Endourol 2001;15: 787–8.

UROLOGIC CLINICS of North America

Urol Clin N Am 34 (2007) 53–59

Urologic Malignancies in Pregnancy

Frances M. Martin, MD, Randall G. Rowland, MD, PhD*

Division of Urology, Department of Surgery, University of Kentucky College of Medicine, University of Kentucky Chandler Medical Center, 800 Rose Street, Room MS-283, Lexington, KY 40536, USA

Cancer is the second leading cause of death in women during reproductive years. Urological tumors occur with an incidence of 1 in 1000 pregnancies. Urologic malignances are rare during pregnancy; therefore, diagnosis and management are problematic. Treatment of tumors of the adrenal gland, kidney, ureter, bladder, and urethra are reviewed.

Testing during pregnancy can uncover incidental tumors, but confounding symptoms during pregnancy can delay the diagnosis of cancer. Urological tumor symptoms, such as pain, hematuria, and hypertension may be mistaken for other, more common conditions such as urinary infection, pyelonephritis, threatened abortion or preeclampsia [1]. Such symptoms warrant a thorough urologic evaluation.

Evaluation for urologic tumors relies upon radiographic testing. In the pregnant patient, the risk to the mother and the fetus must be taken into consideration when diagnostic testing is considered. This issue of the Urologic Clinics of North America also includes an article on urologic radiology in pregnancy, which discusses the issue of fetal radiation risk in detail. There is no proven safe dose of radiation exposure to the fetus [2]. A review article by Loughlin described a relative risk of 1.6 for leukemia and of 3.2 for solid organ cancers in fetuses exposed to 1.6 to 40 mGy radiation dose before delivery [3]. Radiation exposure should be avoided, unless the study will have a major impact on the care of the mother, and the relevant information cannot be obtained in any other way. With modern technology, an accurate

diagnosis usually can be established with ultrasound or MRI.

After establishing a diagnosis, the tumor type and duration of pregnancy determine the treatment options and the timing of therapy. Depending upon the tumor type and stage, therapy may include chemotherapy or surgery. Timing of treatment must be discussed with the patient. Discussion must include the risks of immediate treatment to the health of the fetus and risks of delayed treatment to the mother, such as tumor progression.

Adrenal tumors

Pheochromocytomas during pregnancy are rare, occurring approximately once in every 50,000 term pregnancies [4]. These neuroendocrine tumors arise from chromaffin cells that synthesize, store, and secrete catecholamines and vasoactive peptides. Most tumors arise from an adenoma in one or both adrenal glands. Approximately 10% of pheochromocytomas, however, arise from extra-adrenal locations. Most tumors are sporadic, but 10% are inherited and associated with multiple endocrine neoplasia (MEN) syndromes, von Hippel-Lindau disease, and neurofibromatosis type 1 [5].

Pheochromocytomas typically present with hypertension, headaches, heart palpitations, and hyperhidrosis. Approximately 250 cases of pheochromocytoma during pregnancy have been reported. The severity of presenting symptoms varies from labile hypertension to cardiovascular collapse at delivery. Pheochromocytoma should be suspected in a patient who has severe or fluctuating hypertension, headaches, palpitations, dizziness, nausea, vomiting, visual changes, or

* Corresponding author.

E-mail address: rrowlan@uky.edu (R.G. Rowland).

0094-0143/07/$ - see front matter © 2006 Elsevier Inc. All rights reserved.
doi:10.1016/j.ucl.2006.10.003

congestive heart failure. Unlike preeclampsia, pheochromocytoma usually does not cause proteinuria and is associated with hypertension earlier in pregnancy [6].

Initial testing to diagnose pheochromocytoma may include plasma catecholamine levels; however, 24-hour urine testing is standard. A properly collected 24-hour urine sample is tested for catecholamines and their metabolites: vanilmadelic acid (VMA), metanephrines, normetanephrines, dopamine, epinephrine, and norepinephrine. Elevated levels suggest pheochromocytoma. Provocative testing in pregnant patients is not recommended. The clonidine suppression test and glucagon stimulation test increase the risk of hemodynamic instability and do not add to diagnostic sensitivity and specificity [7].

The tumor may be localized initially by ultrasound, MRI, or CT. MRI is generally the modality of choice, because a bright mass on T2-weighted images distinguishes a pheochromocytoma from incidental adrenal adenomas [8]. Ultrasound may not localize extra-adrenal tumors, and CT exposes the fetus to radiation. Scintigraphy with meta-iodo-benzyl-guanidine (MIBG) is avoided for fetal protection [6].

Definitive treatment of pheochromocytoma is surgical excision. Before surgery, patients must be stabilized medically and prepared for surgery. An alpha blocker, such as phenoxybenzamine, should be initiated at the time of diagnosis. No reported adverse reactions to the fetus have occurred with phenoxybenzamine, which is started at 10 mg orally twice per day and increased every other day by 10 mg and three times per day until blood pressure is controlled within normal ranges. After 1 to 2 weeks of treatment with an alpha-blocker, beta blockers are administered. Selective beta-1 antagonists are preferred, such as atenolol or metoprolol, as propranolol has been associated with intrauterine growth retardation [6]. Beta blockers should be given for several days before planned surgical procedure. Beta blockage never should be attempted before alpha-blockade, because it may lead to unopposed alpha stimulation and result in severe vasoconstriction and possible death [7].

The timing of surgical excision of pheochromocytomas in pregnancy is controversial and depends largely on gestational age at presentation. Early in pregnancy, termination may be offered in combination with mass resection. Surgical outcomes during the first trimester are variable, with risk of fetal death ranging from 20% to 44% [9,10]. If the patient does not want to terminate the pregnancy, and the diagnosis is made in the first trimester or early second trimester, the tumor should be removed as soon as the patient is medically stable with appropriate antiadrenergic blockade. If the diagnosis is made late in the second trimester or in the third trimester, excision may be delayed with medical treatment until the fetus is viable. The delay in surgery may increase the risk of hemorrhage into the tumor, tumor growth, and hypertensive crisis. Delivery should be performed as soon as fetal lung maturity is attained.

The preferred route of delivery is also controversial. In the past, vaginal delivery was associated with higher maternal mortality than caesarian section (31% versus 19%) [11]. Most authors recommend planned caesarian section with concomitant tumor resection to avoid two anesthetic procedures. The safety evidence of laparoscopic surgery during pregnancy is increasing; multiple case reports of laparoscopic adrenalectomy for pheochromocytoma have been reported with no sequelae caused by CO_2 pneumoperitoneum [12].

Before 1970, 25% of pheochromocytomas in pregnant patients were not diagnosed until the patient was in labor. In 1990, 85% of cases were diagnosed before the onset of labor [5]. Higher degree of clinical suspicion and improvements in pharmacologic treatments have reduced maternal mortality from 46% to 4% and fetal mortality from 55% to 15% in the last 15 years. Antenatal diagnosis is a key factor in reducing mortality.

Cortical adenomas

Cortical adrenal tumors may affect cortisol levels. Cushing's syndrome during pregnancy is rare secondary to the suppressive effect of excessive glucocorticord on the reproductive system. Adrenal adenoma is the most common cause of Cushing's syndrome during pregnancy. Blanco and colleagues [13] report hypercortisolism was controlled successfully with metyrapone, which was started at 8 weeks of gestation. At 16 weeks of gestation, a laparoscopic left adrenalectomy was performed. The patient had a normal vaginal delivery at 30 weeks gestation. The infant was a normal virilized male with no apparent teratogenic effects from medical treatment or evidence of adrenal suppression.

Aldosteronomas rarely complicate pregnancy. Patients typically present with preeclampsia and hypokalemia [14]. Medical management, potassium replacement, and adrenalectomy have been reported during pregnancy. Timing of surgery remains controversial, and outcomes are variable.

Incidental tumors of the adrenal gland can be detected during routine ultrasound testing. The natural history of these tumors during pregnancy is unknown. Estrogen during pregnancy may influence the function and proliferation of adrenal cells [15]. Porcaro and colleagues recommend close surveillance on adrenal incidental tumors, as up to 20% may be undetected pheochromocytomas [16].

Renal tumors

Renal cell carcinoma, although rare, is the most common urologic tumor of pregnancy. The most common symptoms at presentation are pain, palpable mass, hematuria, and hypertension [17]. These symptoms in association with pregnancy may delay diagnosis and initially be treated as pre-eclampsia or urinary tract infection. Fortunately, more tumors are being identified during antenatal testing with improvements in ultrasound and prenatal care.

Evaluation for flank pain, hematuria, or renal mass should minimize radiation to the fetus. Ultrasound and urine cytology should be obtained initially. If ultrasound is not sufficient for diagnosis, MRI can identify and differentiate cystic lesions from solid renal cell carcinoma adequately.

Once a suspicious tumor is identified, the standard treatment of most stages of renal carcinoma is radical nephrectomy. The management of cancer during pregnancy must consider the biological behavior of the tumor and the survival rates of the fetus for different gestational ages when timing surgery. Historically, renal carcinomas presented in advanced stages; with increasing incidental renal mass findings on ultrasound, recommendations and timing of treatment may vary. In the first trimester and early second trimester, immediate surgery traditionally is recommended [17,18] despite increased risk of fetal mortality. Late in the second trimester and in the third trimester, fetal lung maturity can be established or improved with antenatal corticosteroids before excision.

Walker and Knight [19] suggest that caesarian section should not automatically be performed at the time of surgery with either a flank incision or laparoscopic nephrectomy. Many case reports describe laparoscopic radical nephrectomy as a safe alternative to open surgery during first, second, or third trimester pregnancies [20,21].

Pregnancy and cancer are the only two biological conditions in which antigenic tissue is tolerated by a normally functioning immune system [17]. There are no studies demonstrating immunodeficiencies in pregnancy that allow for tumor progression, and in most cases the behavior of the tumor is not affected by pregnancy. As recently as 2002, epidemiological studies suggested that hormonal influences play a role in the development of renal cell carcinoma [22,23]. Lambe and colleagues observed a positive association between parity and renal cell carcinoma. In their study, for each additional birth, a woman had an associated 15% increase in risk of developing renal cell carcinoma. The authors report that their evidence needs further investigation since increased incidence also was associated with increasing body mass index (BMI), hypertension, and diabetes.

Benign renal tumors

The second most common type of renal mass identified during pregnancy is angiomyolipoma (AML). AML is a benign fibro-fatty tumor typically associated with tuberous sclerosis. Data show that approximately half of all patients with AML do not have tuberous sclerosis. These tumors are usually single and unilateral and composed of adipose tissue, smooth muscle, and thick-walled blood vessels.

Although most AMLs are asymptomatic, they may become worrisome or life-threatening secondary to bleeding. Patients with AML may present with hematuria, flank pain, mass, or retroperitoneal hemorrhage. Spontaneous rupture of AML is rare, but associated with size larger than 4 cm. Sporadic reports of massive retroperitoneal hemorrhage and shock during pregnancy have been described [24].

Diagnosis of AML typically is based upon ultrasound or CT findings showing a hyperechoic mass and demonstration of fat within the tumor. MRI or angiography also may be diagnostic. MRI avoids high-dose radiation. Angiography may provide diagnostic value and therapeutic treatment of bleeding.

Treatment options include excision, either laparoscopic or open, with total or partial nephrectomy, cryoablation, radiofrequency ablation, or embolization [25]. Therapy for diagnosed AML ideally is performed once the tumor becomes 4 cm in size before pregnancy. AML not diagnosed until pregnancy may be treated conservatively with observation if the patient is asymptomatic or remains hemodynamically stable [26]. Conservative management and vaginal delivery following a ruptured AML have been reported [27]. If bleeding persists or results in hemodynamic instability, selective angioembolization with alcohol, coils, or gel–foam may provide nephron-sparing treatment and can be performed with minimal radiation exposure to the fetus [25]. Lewis and Palmer [24] presented a case report in which an unstable patient in the third trimester underwent caesarian section followed by immediate nephrectomy for bleeding that resulted in a healthy neonate and full recovery of the patient.

Ureteral tumors

Transitional cell carcinoma of the ureter is rare, and two case reports exist in English in the literature. The first patient was 42 years old and was diagnosed before pregnancy, but refused medical or surgical treatment. She presented 24 days after delivery with widely metastatic disease and sepsis [28]. The second presented with flank pain and hematuria. She required nephrectomy during pregnancy secondary to rupture of the renal pelvis. She delivered a healthy infant later, but required subsequent ureterectomy [29].

Benign tumors of the ureter exist. Malakoplakia is an inflammatory condition presenting as a plaque or a nodule that usually affects the genitourinary tract. Microscopically, malakoplakia is characterized by the presence of foamy histiocytes with distinctive basophilic inclusions, which are known as Michaelis-Gutmann bodies. This microscopic finding is believed to result from the inadequate killing of bacteria by macrophages or monocytes that exhibit defective phagolysosomal activity. Partially digested bacteria accumulate in monocytes or macrophages and lead to the deposition of calcium and iron on residual bacterial glycolipid. Malakoplakia occurs more frequently in immunocompromised patients and does not show an increased incidence during pregnancy. Treatment consists of prolonged antibiotic therapy.

Bladder tumors

Bladder cancer during pregnancy is rare and can consist of transitional cell carcinoma, adenocarcinoma, or squamous cell carcinoma.

Squamous cell carcinoma is associated with bilharzial infections with *Schistosoma haematobium* and is rare in the United States. In Egypt, it occurs more frequently in younger patients. Therefore, bilharzial bladder cancer often is encountered during pregnancy [30]. Adenocarcinoma is rare, comprising less than 2% of all bladder neoplasms, but it has been reported during pregnancy. Typically patients present with urgency, frequency, and occasionally hematuria.

The presenting symptoms for transitional cell carcinoma and adenocarcinoma of the bladder are similar. Fewer than 50 cases of nonbilharzial bladder cancers have been reported. Because bladder cancer is so rare, the symptoms are frequently misleading and delay diagnosis.

The evaluation of a pregnant patient who has bleeding must include a urinalysis and urine culture obtained by catheterization to distinguish between urinary and vaginal bleeding [31]. Although 81% of women with bladder cancer presented with hematuria, 22% initially were misdiagnosed with vaginal bleeding. If urinary tract infection is confirmed, treatment with appropriate antibiotics should be followed by repeat urinalysis. If hematuria persists with no evidence of infection, the patient should be evaluated by ultrasound and cystoscopy [31].

Ultrasound is used to diagnose calculi or renal tumors, but it is not sufficient to adequately evaluate the bladder. Only 52% of bladder tumors were diagnosed on ultrasound of the reported cases [31]. Therefore, cystoscopy is necessary and may be performed as an office procedure. No complications have been reported with flexible endoscopy under local anesthesia during pregnancy [32]. Of note, urine cytology may be helpful to evaluate for cancer, but negative results are frequent in the presence of low-grade carcinomas, and it cannot postpone or replace cystoscopy.

Once a suspicious area or obvious abnormality is identified, transurethral resection of the lesion is recommended. In general, treatment for bladder carcinoma during pregnancy should not differ from treatment for the general population [31]. Resection of the lesion can be performed under regional or general anesthesia. Few complications have been reported during transurethral resection, but changes of bladder conformation during pregnancy must be considered [33].

Once the staging of the cancer is complete, discussion of treatment options must consider the stage and type of tumor, stage of pregnancy, and patient's preference. For low-risk tumors, defined as a single lesion less than 3 cm, pathological stage pTaG1, initial resection should be followed by cystoscopy every 3 months with a good prognosis for patient and fetus [31].

For intermediate-risk tumors consisting of multifocal tumors, greater than 3 cm, pathological stage pTa-1, G1-2, recurrence is more likely. The standard treatment is complete resection followed by subsequent resection in 4 to 6 weeks. In nonpregnant patients, the standard would include intravesical therapy for recurrence. Mitomycin C, thiotepa, and doxorubicin are avoided during pregnancy, although studies are unclear on absorption and teratotoxicity. Wax and colleagues [34] reported the only case of BCG vaccine administration during pregnancy. The patient had progression from a solitary tumor before pregnancy to multifocal carcinoma in situ (CIS) during pregnancy. She underwent two 6-week courses of BCG and subsequently delivered a healthy neonate at term. Postpartum, the patient required additional resection and instillation of BCG and interferon. If possible, chemotherapeutic agents should be started after delivery with preference for repeat transurethral resection of recurrent lesions.

For high-risk tumors, including CIS and pT1G3, treatment consists of resection of all lesions followed by a second procedure at 4 to 6 weeks. When possible, induction of delivery should proceed as soon as fetal maturation is confirmed, and intravesical therapy should be initiated after delivery. For muscle-invasive tumors and adenocarcinoma, the treatment depends upon the stage of pregnancy. Prognosis is poor, and several authors recommend termination of pregnancy if diagnosed in the first trimester [35]. If the tumor is detected late in the second trimester or the third trimester, cesarean section may be performed at 28 weeks of gestation followed by immediate radical cystectomy [32]. Because the occurrence of invasive bladder cancer is rare, no consensus exists, and each case must have a tailored treatment plan.

Gestational trophoblastic disease metastatic to the bladder and extra-adrenal paragangliomas have been reported. Also, benign lesion of the bladder may present during pregnancy, such as leiomyoma or fibroepithelial polyps. These lesions must be evaluated as in nonpregnant patients.

In reviewing the literature, studies have weakly supported that parity and age at first pregnancy may decrease the risk of developing bladder cancer [36]. The authors suggest that hormonal changes during pregnancy may be protective against oncogenesis. Further investigation is necessary before definite information on any link between hormonal changes and bladder cancer risk can be addressed.

Urethral tumors

Carcinoma of the urethra is a rare lesion presenting as squamous cell carcinoma, transitional cell carcinoma, or adenocarcinoma. Severino and colleagues [37] presented a case report in 1977 of urethral adenocarcinoma during pregnancy. The pregnancy was continued to term and delivered vaginally. The patient subsequently was treated with radiotherapy and urethrectomy and had at least 7 years of disease-free survival.

Benign tumors of the urethra may increase in size during pregnancy. Such lesions include urethral caruncle, prolapse, polyp, granuloma gravidarum, and leiomyoma [38]. Three urethral leiomyomas have been found in pregnancy. Kesari and colleagues [39] described estrogen receptors stained by immunohistochemistry throughout the leiomyoma, suggesting a possible etiology for its occurrence during pregnancy. Treatment consists of simple surgical excision [40].

Summary

Tumors do occur during pregnancy in all portions of the urologic tract. Fortunately, urologic malignancies are rare during pregnancy. Unfortunately, the presenting symptoms often are misdiagnosed because of confounding symptoms of pregnancy such as hypertension, bleeding, recurrent urinary tract infections, and hydronephrosis of pregnancy. On the other hand, testing and ultrasonography for pregnancy can discover incidental tumors that must be addressed. Evaluation for tumors must include radiological testing. The testing chosen should provide the most information while exposing the fetus to minimal amounts of radiation. Diagnosing malignancies before delivery can be life-saving for the patient and improve survival of the fetus. A high index of suspicion helps prevent missing these tumors. Depending upon the tumor type and stage and gestational age, treatment options are highly variable. All options should be discussed with the patient, and individual treatment plans should be devised based upon risks of immediate therapy versus delayed treatment.

References

[1] Hendry WF. Management of urological tumors in pregnancy. Br J Urol 1997;80(Suppl 1):24–8.

[2] Mole RH. Childhood cancer after prenatal exposure to diagnostic x-ray examinations in Britain. Br J Cancer 1990;62:152–68.

[3] Loughlin KR. The Management of Urological Malignancies during Pregnancy. Br J Urol 1995;76: 639–44.

[4] Potts JM, Larrimer J. Pheochromocytoma in a pregnant patient. J Fam Pract 1994;22:1–10.

[5] Lyman DJ. Paroxysmal hypertension, pheochromocytoma, and pregnancy. J Am Board Fam Pract 2002;15(2):153–8.

[6] Mannelli M, Bemporad D. Diagnosis and management of pheochromocytoma during pregnancy. J Endocrinol Invest 2002;25(6):567–71.

[7] Bailit J, Neerhof M. Diagnosis and management of pheochromocytoma in pregnancy: a case report. Am J Perinatol 1998;15(4):259–62.

[8] Langerman A, Schneider JA, Ward RP. Pheochromocytoma storm presenting as cardiovascular collapse at term pregnancy. Rev Cardiovasc Med 2004;5(4):226–30.

[9] Keely E. Endocrine causes of hypertension in pregnancy—when to start looking for zebras. Semin Perinatol 1998;22:471–84.

[10] Ahlawat SK, Jain S, Kumari S, et al. Pheochromocytoma associated with pregnancy: case report and review of the literature. Obstet Gynecol Surv 1999; 54:728–37.

[11] Schenker JG, Granat M. Phaeochromocytoma and pregnancy—an updated appraisal. Aust N Z J Obstet Gynaecol 1982;22:1–10.

[12] Kim PTW, Kreisman S, Vaughn R, et al. Laparoscopic adrenalectomy for pheochromocytoma in pregnancy. Can J Surg 2006;49(1):62–3.

[13] Blanco C, Maqueda E, Rubio JA, et al. Cushing's syndrome during pregnancy secondary to adrenal adenoma; metyrapone treatment and laparoscopic adrenalectomy. J Endocrinol Invest 2006;29(2): 164–7.

[14] Okawa TAK, Hashimoto T, Fujimori K, et al. Diagnosis and management of primary aldosteronism in pregnancy: case report and review of the literature. Am J Perinatol 2002;19(1):31–6.

[15] Fallo F, Pezzi V, Sonino N, et al. Adrenal incidentaloma in pregnancy: clinical, molecular, and immunohistochemical findings. J Endocrinol Invest 2005;28(5):459–63.

[16] Porcaro ABNG, Ficarra V, D'Amico A, et al. Incidental adrenal pheochromocytoma. Report on 5 operated patients and update of the literature. Arch Ital Urol Androl 2003;75(4):217–25.

[17] Gladman MA, MacDonald D, Webster JJ. Renal cell carcinoma in pregnancy. J R Soc Med 2002; 95(4):199–201.

[18] Fynn J, Venyo AK. Renal cell carcinoma presenting as hypertension in pregnancy. J Obstet Gynaecol 2004;24(7):821–2.

[19] Walker JL, Knight EL. Renal cell carcinoma in pregnancy. Cancer 1986;58(10):2343–7.

[20] O'Connor JP, Biyani CS, Taylor J, et al. Laparoscopic nephrectomy for renal cell carcinoma during pregnancy. J Endourol 2004;18(9):871–4.

[21] Sainsbury DC, Dorkin TJ, MacPhail S, et al. Laparoscopic radical nephrectomy in first-trimester pregnancy. Urology 2004;64(6):1231. e7–8.

[22] Lambe M, Lindblad P, Wuu J, et al. Pregnancy and risk of renal cell cancer: a population-based study in Sweden. Br J Cancer 2002;86(9):1425–9.

[23] Mydlo JH, Chawla S, Dorn S, et al. Renal cancer and pregnancy in two different female cohorts. Can J Urol 2002;9(5):1634–6.

[24] Lewis EL, Palmer JM. Renal angiomyolipoma and massive retroperitoneal hemorrhage during pregnancy. West J Med 1985;143(5):675–6.

[25] Morales JP, Georganas M, Khan MS, et al. Embolization of a bleeding renal angiomyolipoma in pregnancy: case report and review. Cardiovasc Intervent Radiol 2005;28(2):265–8.

[26] Khaitan A, Hemal AK, Seth A, et al. Management of renal angiomyolipoma in complex clinical situations. Urol Int 2001;67(1):28–33.

[27] Tanaka M, Kyo S, Inoue M, et al. Conservative management and vaginal delivery following ruptured renal angiomyolipoma. Obstet Gynecol 2001; 98:932–3.

[28] Pasini J, Mokos I, Delmis J, et al. Disseminated ureteral carcinoma discovered in a woman patient at childbirth. Eur J Obstet Gynecol Reprod Biol 2005;121(2):252–3.

[29] Texter JH Jr, Bellinger M, Kawamoto E, et al. Persistent hematuria during pregnancy. J Urol 1980; 123(1):84–8.

[30] Badawy S, Karim M. Bilharzial carcinoma of the bladder with pregnancy and labor. Int Surg 1971; 56(6):434–7.

[31] Spahn M, Bader P, Westermann D, et al. Bladder carcinoma during pregnancy. Urol Int 2005;74(2): 153–9.

[32] Wax JR, Pinette MG, Blackstone J, et al. Nonbilharzial bladder carcinoma complicating pregnancy: review of the literature. Obstet Gynecol Surv 2002; 57(4):236–44.

[33] Gupta NP, Dorairajan LN. Transurethral resection of a bladder tumor in pregnancy: a report of 2 cases. Int Urogynecol J Pelvic Floor Dysfunct 1997;8(4): 230–2.

[34] Wax JR, Ross J, Marotto L, et al. Nonbilharzial bladder carcinoma complicating pregnancy–treatment with bacille Calmette-Guerin. Am J Obstet Gynecol 2002;187(1):239–40.

[35] Loughlin KR, Ng B. Bladder cancer during pregnancy. Br J Urol 1995;75(3):421–2.

[36] Cantor KP, Lynch CF, Johnson D. Bladder cancer, parity, and age at first birth. Cancer Causes Control 1992;3(1):57–62.

[37] Severino LJ, Brockunier A Jr, Davidian MM. Adenocarcinoma of the urethra during pregnancy: report of a case. Obstet Gynecol 1977;50(Suppl Jr): 22S–3S.

[38] Rao AR, Motiwala H. Urethral hemangioma. Urology 2005;65(5):1000.

[39] Kesari D, Gemer O, Segal S, et al. Estrogen receptors in a urethral leiomyoma presenting in pregnancy. Int J Gynaecol Obstet 1994;47(1):59–60.

[40] Shield DE, Weiss RM. Leiomyoma of the female urethra. J Urol 1973;109(3):430–1.

ELSEVIER
SAUNDERS

Urol Clin N Am 34 (2007) 61–69

UROLOGIC
CLINICS
of North America

Pregnancy and Interstitial Cystitis/Painful Bladder Syndrome

Deborah R. Erickson, MD[a],*, Kathleen J. Propert, ScD[b]

[a]Division of Urology, Department of Surgery, University of Kentucky College of Medicine,
University of Kentucky Chandler Medical Center, 800 Rose Street, Room MS-269,
Lexington, KY 40536, USA
[b]Department of Biostatistics and Epidemiology, University of Pennsylvania School of Medicine, 6th Floor,
Blockley Hall, 423 Guardian Drive, Philadelphia, PA 19104, USA

Introduction

Interstitial cystitis (IC) is a syndrome that includes pelvic or perineal pain, urgency to urinate, and frequent voiding both day and night. For decades, clinicians and researchers have tried to establish a precise definition for IC, but no specific definition has been widely accepted. Recently the International Continence Society introduced a new term, painful bladder syndrome (PBS), which is defined as "the complaint of suprapubic pain related to bladder filling, accompanied by other symptoms such as increased daytime and nighttime frequency, in the absence of proven urinary infection or other obvious pathology" [1]. PBS and IC thus have many similarities. However, the two are not identical; for example, pain is required for the definition of PBS, but some IC patients complain only of urgency and frequency but deny pain. Because of the significant overlap between PBS and IC, this article uses the term PBS/IC as a general term. For descriptions of the previous literature, this article uses the same nomenclature that was used in the cited article.

Proposed causes of painful bladder syndrome/interstitial cystitis

Many different causes have been proposed for PBS/IC, and some of them may overlap. A detailed discussion of the various causes and the

* Corresponding author.
E-mail address: dreric2@email.uky.edu
(D.R. Erickson).

evidence for and against each one is beyond the scope of this article. The major theories are described briefly, in terms of their potential relevance to pregnancy.

The most commonly stated theory is that the bladder urothelium is deficient. Urothelial deficiency may be the primary problem in PBS/IC, or it may be secondary to another process, such as bladder inflammation. The factors that affect normal and abnormal urothelium are not completely understood, but both estrogen and progesterone have been reported to stimulate growth of cultured (ureteral) urothelial cells [2,3]. The hormonal changes during pregnancy thus may affect the bladder urothelium. Estrogen and progesterone also influence growth factors, such as nerve growth factor, epidermal growth factor (EGF) and heparin-binding EGF-like growth factor [2–4]. All three of these factors have been shown to be altered in the urine or bladder of IC patients [5–7]. The hormonal changes of pregnancy may influence IC symptoms by modulating the effects of these growth factors.

Another main theory is that mast cells are activated in the bladder, releasing histamine and other mediators that cause pain and inflammation. Hormonal changes of pregnancy might influence PBS/IC because, in general, mast cell activation is augmented by estrogen. Specific to IC, human bladder mast cells express estrogen receptors, and these cells were found to be more numerous in IC bladders than control bladders (reviewed in [8]).

Another main theory is that PBS/IC is an allergic or autoimmune process in the bladder.

This theory suggests another way that hormonal changes in pregnancy may affect IC, because gonadal steroids are well known to modulate inflammation. In general, estrogen enhances inflammation and androgens and progesterone are suppressors [9]. However, to our knowledge, no studies have specifically addressed the roles of gonadal steroids on bladder inflammation in PBS/IC, other than the effects on mast cells as mentioned above.

A more recent theory is that altered bladder innervation may cause or perpetuate the symptoms of IC. This theory suggests another way that pregnancy may influence PBS/IC symptoms. Gonadal hormones have many effects on the central and peripheral nervous systems [10,11]. Pregnancy also is associated with increased pain threshold [12].

Painful bladder syndrome/interstitial cystitis symptoms during pregnancy

The previous section discussed several possible mechanisms by which pregnancy might affect PBS/IC pathophysiology. However, no studies have directly examined these or any other aspects of PBS/IC during pregnancy, except for symptoms alone. Most of the studies on symptoms were retrospective.

The Interstitial Cystitis Association conducted a patient survey about symptoms and pregnancy in 1989 [13]. Patients who described their baseline IC symptoms as "mild" experienced worsening symptoms during pregnancy, which persisted up to 6 months after delivery. In contrast, patients who described their IC as "severe" had a significant improvement in symptoms during the second trimester, which lasted up to 6 months after delivery or for the duration of breastfeeding. IC outcome was not affected by the mode of delivery (vaginal versus cesarean section).

Pregnancy questions were also included in the Interstitial Cystitis database (ICDB) study, a multicenter prospective observational study sponsored by the National Institute of Diabetes and Digestive and Kidney Diseases [14]. Patients were followed for up to 3 years and extensive data were collected. One question was the relationship of symptom onset to pregnancy. Of 582 women in the study, 144 (25%) had never been pregnant. For those 433 who had been pregnant at least once and provided data on pregnancy and symptoms, 274 (63%) said their symptom onset had

no relation to pregnancy, 95 (22%) had symptom onset before the first pregnancy, 30 (7%) had symptom onset during a pregnancy, and 34 (8%) had symptom onset during the first 6 months after a delivery. The patients also were asked whether their IC symptoms improved during any pregnancy. Only 7% of the evaluable patients answered yes. The ICDB study did not analyze whether symptom relief during pregnancy was associated with initial symptom severity or other clinical features.

Both of the above studies were limited by their retrospective nature with respect to associations with pregnancy, and symptom assessment during pregnancy was based on patient recall. To date, only one prospective study of IC during pregnancy has been published [15]. The study included 12 patients who had IC who had glomerulations on cystoscopy and whose bladder biopsies showed chronic inflammation with or without mast cells. Eleven patients had a course of dimethylsulfoxide (DMSO) (every two weeks for 12 weeks) and all had symptom remission. One patient declined DMSO and the authors did not specify how her symptom remission was accomplished. Pregnancy occurred 6 months to 5 years after the DMSO treatment. Nine patients continued to have good symptom remission throughout pregnancy. The other 3 had worsening symptoms, and 2 patients terminated the pregnancy because of severe symptoms. Because this small group of patients was more homogeneous than the general IC population, with all patients having chronic inflammation on bladder biopsy and good remission after DMSO, it is unclear how the results of this study apply to the general PBS/IC population.

Painful bladder syndrome/interstitial cystitis treatments in pregnancy

General considerations

The United States Food and Drug Administration established a classification system for safety of drug use in pregnancy. The categories and their definitions are described in this issue in the article on pharmaceutic agents and pregnancy. Briefly, A: adequate human studies showed no increased risk to the fetus; B: animal studies showed no increased risk, or animal studies showed an increased risk but adequate human studies showed no increased risk; C: there are no adequate human studies, and animal studies either showed an increased risk or have not been done;

D: human studies showed increased risk, but the drug can be used if the benefits clearly outweigh the risks; X: definite evidence of fetal abnormalities, should not be used during pregnancy.

A wide variety of drugs, both oral and intravesical, are used to treat PBS/IC. This plethora of treatments has evolved because no single treatment is universally effective. For the nonpregnant patient, the usual strategy is to try different treatments empirically. Treatments that work for a given patient are continued, and ineffective or intolerable treatments are stopped. For the pregnant patient, the fetal risks are weighed against the degree of symptom relief provided by a specific treatment. If she is already using the treatment, then she knows how effective that treatment is for her. If she wants to try a new treatment while pregnant, the risks are weighed against the probability of that treatment giving good symptom relief. When making these decisions, it should be kept in mind that the baseline risk for fetal malformations is approximately 2% to 4% [16]. This section discusses the pregnancy risks for the most commonly used PBS/IC treatments.

Pentosan polysulfate

Pentosan polysulfate (PPS) is listed as a category B drug [17]. In cultured mouse embryos, reversible limb bud abnormalities occurred when PPS (1 mg/mL) was added to the culture medium. In contrast, for animals given IV doses of 7.5 to 15 mg/kg, there was no evidence of impaired fertility or fetal harm. A possible explanation for this discrepancy is that PPS may not cross the placenta. This explanation has not been formally tested to our knowledge, but PPS is structurally similar to heparin, and heparin is believed not to cross the placenta and to be safe in pregnancy [16]. Also, because of its large size and high negative charge, PPS has low absorption from the GI tract [17,18]. Approximately 3% of an oral dose of PPS is absorbed, so the human daily oral dose of 300 mg/day would be equivalent to about 9 mg IV per day (for a 70-kg person, about 0.13 mg/kg/day), which is much less than the doses used in the animal studies described above.

To our knowledge, no published studies directly evaluated the fetal risk for human patients taking PPS. However, the factors described above suggest that PPS is likely to be safe. A patient who is experiencing significant symptom relief with PPS therefore might choose to continue it during pregnancy. Conversely, as a new treatment to try

during pregnancy, PPS has disadvantages. It usually takes 3 to 6 months for symptom relief to occur, and the response rate is highly variable. In five placebo-controlled trials, the response rates ranged from 28% to 63%, and two of the trials concluded that PPS was not more effective than placebo (for review see [18]).

Amitriptyline

Amitriptyline is listed by the manufacturer as a category C drug [19]. It crosses the human placenta [20] and had adverse fetal effects in some animal models but not others [19,21]. In studies comparing different antidepressants for genotoxicity, amitriptyline was not genotoxic but it did inhibit apoptosis, so it might affect fetal development by that mechanism [22]. There are sporadic reports of malformations in infants whose mothers took amitriptyline during pregnancy (with or without other drugs) [16,19,21]. However, in large studies, amitriptyline exposure during pregnancy did not increase the incidence of fetal abnormalities, nor did it affect the development of the young children in follow-up [16,19,23–26]. The literature contains case reports of withdrawal symptoms in neonates whose mothers were taking other tricyclic antidepressants (clomipramine, imipramine, desipramine; reviewed in [23]). To our knowledge there are no such reports for amitriptyline. Several textbooks state that amitriptyline is relatively safe in pregnancy [19,27,28]. Also, because of the long experience with its use, it may be preferred over newer antidepressants during pregnancy [19].

In view of the overall experience with amitriptyline, it seems to have low risk. If a patient is already taking it and has significant symptom relief, she might choose to continue it during pregnancy. If a patient wants to try it as a new treatment, she should consider the results of placebo-controlled trials using amitriptyline for PBS/IC. To date only one such trial has been published [29]. With response defined as at least 30% improvement in symptom score, response rates were 42% for amitriptyline and 12.5% for placebo.

Hydroxyzine

Hydroxyzine is listed as a category C drug [30]. When given to animals in high doses (above the human therapeutic range), it was teratogenic in mice and rats but not rabbits [30,31]. For humans, the data are summarized in a recent review by

Gilbert and colleagues [32] from the Motherisk program at the Hospital for Sick Children in Toronto. In three studies, the relative risk for fetal malformations with hydroxyzine ranged from 1.4 to 3.07. This was greater than the relative risks for any of the other antihistamines in their review. Another consideration is that withdrawal symptoms have been reported in four infants born to mothers taking hydroxyzine late in pregnancy (reviewed in [33]).

The literature to date contains only one placebo-controlled trial of hydroxyzine as an IC treatment [34]. In that study, symptom response was defined as "moderate" or "marked" improvement on a patient-reported global response assessment, using a seven-point centered scale. The response rates were 31% for hydroxyzine and 20% for placebo ($P = .26$). With this low response rate, the benefit of trying hydroxyzine as a new treatment during pregnancy might not outweigh the fetal risks described above. Conversely, a patient who already takes it with good results might decide that the benefits of continuing do outweigh the risks. Such a patient could also consider changing to cetirizine. Cetirizine is category B, it was not teratogenic in animal studies, and in two human studies the relative risks of fetal malformations were 1.15 and 1.22, respectively [32,35]. The patient is likely to ask whether cetirizine will improve her symptoms as well as hydroxyzine. The answer is unknown. The first thought is that is should work just as well, because it is an active metabolite of hydroxyzine and also a histamine receptor antagonist, but less sedating than the parent drug [36]. However, antihistamines are not just histamine receptor antagonists. They have a variety of other antiinflammatory and analgesic effects [37–40]. It is unknown which of these effects is responsible for the benefit of hydroxyzine in any given PBS/IC patient, and it is unknown whether the beneficial effects are stronger, weaker or similar for cetirizine compared with hydroxyzine.

Intravesical dimethylsulfoxide

DMSO is listed at category C [41]. It was teratogenic in several animal models when given intraperitoneally or topically at doses of 2 to 12 g/kg, but not when given topically to rabbits at 1.1 g/kg (the 50-mL dose used for IC treatment contains 27 g DMSO, or 0.39 g/kg in a 70-kg person) [41]. To our knowledge there is no published experience with DMSO and human pregnancy.

A PubMed search with these terms identified several articles, but they focused on the use of DMSO as a preservative for frozen embryos or cord blood cells. In theory, DMSO could have many systemic effects because of its ability to dissolve lipids and increase permeability of cell membranes [42]. An important example in adults is that DMSO can cause lens opacification [41]. Given these considerations and the virtually nonexistent human data, it is prudent to avoid DMSO during pregnancy. However, a patient who has already achieved a good remission from DMSO is likely to maintain remission without further DMSO treatments during pregnancy [15].

Intravesical heparin

Because of its large size and high negative charge, heparin is unlikely to be absorbed from the bladder after intravesical administration. However, even systemic heparin is considered to be safe in pregnancy, since it is thought not to cross the placenta [16]. The only apparent risk of intravesical heparin during pregnancy is the risk for bacteriuria from passing the catheter. A patient who has achieved good results with intravesical heparin will probably choose to continue it during pregnancy. As a new treatment, the response rate is difficult to predict because there are no placebo-controlled trials published to our knowledge.

Intravesical lidocaine

Absorption of intravesical lidocaine is pH-dependent because the acid form is ionized and unlikely to cross the bladder epithelium [43]. The pH of lidocaine for injection is approximately 6.5 [44]. Because greater than 90% of the lidocaine is in the acid form at this pH, its absorption from the bladder should be minimal [43]. As expected, several studies with intravesical lidocaine doses from 400 to 1000 mg reported serum levels as "negligible" or less than 0.2 mcg/mL (reviewed in [44]; also see [45]). However, two case reports described higher serum levels. One case involved a patient who had severe ulcerative IC and a cystometric capacity of 50 mL, who received 200 mg lidocaine in 40 mL saline for 1 hour twice a day [46]. The peak serum lidocaine concentration was 1.6 mcg/mL (the therapeutic range is 1.5 to 5 mcg/mL) [43]. In this case, the increased absorption was probably attributable to the patient's severe epithelial dysfunction with ulcerative IC, combined with the high filling volume (80% of the patient's functional capacity) and long dwell time. (After 2 weeks of this treatment the patient had complete pain relief and improved frequency.) The other case involved a 2.5-year-old girl who had refractory bladder spasms on the first day after bilateral ureteral reimplants [47]. Fifty mL of 2% lidocaine was instilled through her Foley catheter and left 15 minutes. Five minutes later she had a seizure and her serum lidocaine level was toxic at 7.9 mcg/mL. The increased absorption was attributed to high intravesical pressure during bladder spasms.

In contrast to the acid form, the base form of lidocaine is nonionized and lipid soluble, so it does get systemically absorbed from the bladder. In a solution with pH 7.4, 29% of lidocaine is in the base form. At pH 8.0, 61% is in the base form [41]. Henry and coworkers [43] tested the absorption of alkalinized intravesical lidocaine. In healthy volunteers, they instilled 4 to 6 mg/kg lidocaine, immediately followed by 20 mL 8.4% sodium bicarbonate, into the bladder for a 1-hour dwell time. They followed serum levels at intervals from 30 to 180 minutes after instillation. For each subject, the highest serum level occurred at the first blood draw (ie, at 30 minutes). These levels ranged from 0.66 to 1.71 mcg/mL. They also tested patients who had IC using a slightly modified protocol with 5 mg/kg lidocaine followed by 10 mL 8.4% sodium bicarbonate. Again, the highest serum concentrations were at the 30-minute time point and they ranged from 0.2 to 2.0 mcg/mL. Both volunteers and patients had bladder or urethral discomfort after voiding the solution. The discomfort lasted 1 to 3 hours in the volunteers and hours to days in the patients who had IC.

Parsons [48] recently described a therapeutic cocktail for IC including 8 mL lidocaine, 3 mL 8.4% sodium bicarbonate, and 40,000 units of heparin. The initial lidocaine concentration was 1% (ie, 80 mg per dose), but patients who did not get relief with this were changed to 2% (160 mg). Serum lidocaine levels were not measured, so it is unknown how much lidocaine was absorbed.

If lidocaine does get absorbed systemically, it rapidly crosses the placenta, reaching fetal serum concentrations 0.5 to 1.3 times the maternal concentration [49]. The effects of lidocaine on the fetus are not well defined. Lidocaine is listed as category B and caused no fetal harm when given to pregnant rats [49]. However, most human studies are about use of lidocaine as an anesthetic for labor and delivery, not about chronic use during pregnancy. If lidocaine is used as a PBS/IC treatment during pregnancy, therefore, the safest choice would be to instill non-alkalinized lidocaine and avoid the issue of systemic absorption. The disadvantage is that non-alkalinized lidocaine may not relieve pain as effectively, because of its lower epithelial penetration. If the patient gets relief only from the alkalinized form, measuring the serum levels after instillation may help the patient and clinician to adjust the dose and optimally balance the risks versus benefits.

Intravesical corticosteroids

Systemic corticosteroids are teratogenic in humans and animals. They are listed as category D in the first trimester and category C thereafter [50]. However, a recent study noted that in humans, the main fetal anomaly associated with maternal corticosteroid use was cleft lip or palate, and the risk was increased from a baseline of about 1/1000 to about 3/1000 [51]. Of course, systemic corticosteroids are not used to treat PBS/IC. Intravesical corticosteroids are used, and their absorption from the bladder has not been described in any publications to our knowledge. One study tested absorption of hydrocortisone from ileal neobladders. A total of 2000 mg of hydrocortisone was instilled and blood samples were tested before, 1 hour after, and 2 hours after instillation. The plasma concentrations were two to five times the physiologic levels [52]. However, since the absorptive capabilities of the bladder and bowel are different, these results cannot be directly extrapolated to intravesical instillation. With this lack of knowledge, and the lack of placebo-controlled trials, it is impossible to give accurate advice about starting intravesical corticosteroids during pregnancy. If a patient is already using this treatment with good results, she may believe that the benefits outweigh the risks, especially after the first trimester when palate formation is complete.

Sacral nerve stimulation

Sacral nerve stimulators should not be placed during pregnancy. If a patient has a stimulator already in place, the Medtronic company recommends that she turn it off for the entire pregnancy, because the effects of sacral nerve stimulation on the fetus are completely unknown.

Is painful bladder syndrome/interstitial cystitis hereditary?

A pregnant woman who has PBS/IC may be concerned about the risk for passing on the condition to her child. At this time, because the causes of PBS/IC are still unknown, it is not possible to answer this question precisely (unless she is a member of a unique kindred described later). Epidemiologic studies are hampered by the lack of a well-established clinical definition for IC. Results of different studies may vary, depending on how IC is diagnosed or defined. Studies that ask about IC symptoms (as opposed to a clinical diagnosis) also have variable results because of different symptom questionnaires being used and different cutpoints being applied.

Is there a familial predisposition for PBS/IC? A good way to answer this question would be to compare a sample of PBS/IC patients' first-degree relatives with a sample from the general population, using the same diagnostic criteria or symptom questionnaires for both groups. To our knowledge this has never been done, so the closest approximation is described below.

The first question is: what are the prevalences of diagnosed IC, or PBS/IC symptoms, in the general population? These figures have been estimated in several recent population-based studies from various regions in the United States. For IC diagnosis, the prevalences per 100,000 women were 45, 60, 114, and 197, respectively [53–55]. For PBS/IC symptoms, the prevalences among women were 6.2% to 11.2%, 0.6% to 12.6%, and 31%, respectively [56–58]. The next question is: are these prevalences different for family members of patients who have IC? Warren and colleagues [59] mailed a survey to more than 10,000 patients who had IC, including questions about their family members. Twenty-two percent of the patients returned the survey, giving a data set of 5802 first-degree relatives of patients who had IC. Of these relatives, approximately 1.5% were described as having "confirmed" IC and approximately 12% had symptoms of IC. The prevalence of diagnosed IC was increased compared with that of the general population, but the data are still re-assuring because more than 98% of the relatives did not have an IC diagnosis. Regarding symptoms, the 12% prevalence seen in the IC relatives is comparable to the recently reported prevalences in the general population.

Approaching the question from a different direction, Koziol and colleagues [60] administered questionnaires to 565 patients who had IC and 171 volunteers who did not have IC. One of the questions was whether or not any family members had IC. 16.3% of patients and 17.3% of controls answered yes. In an interim analysis of the ICDB,

5.4% of patients reported having a family member who had IC, but this database did not include a non-IC control group [14].

Overall, population studies suggest that the prevalence of IC may be increased among relatives of patients who have IC, but even so, most of these relatives do not have IC. This finding suggests that IC is sporadic in most cases. However, occasionally one encounters families that have multiple members with IC. For example, the survey by Warren and coworkers [59] found six families in which three members had IC (eg, three sisters, or grandmother, mother, and daughter). In these families there may be a genetic predisposition for IC. To investigate this theory further, the twin pairs in this survey were analyzed [61]. The survey included 32 patients who had "probable" or "confirmed" IC and who also had a living twin. For the 8 patients who had identical twins, 5 of the co-twins had "probable" or "confirmed" IC. In contrast, for the 26 patients who had dizygotic twins, none of the co-twins had "probable" or "confirmed" IC. These findings suggest that IC has a multifactorial cause, with genetic susceptibility as one factor.

A case report and abstract described four Bulgarian families that had IC inherited in an autosomal dominant pattern [62,63]. In these families, the child of an IC patient has approximately a 50% chance of developing IC. This case is obviously different from the usual situation in the United States. However, it is valuable to analyze these families and identify the specific genetic alterations associated with IC, because knowledge of these genes may shed more light on the cause of IC in the general population also.

Summary and key points

PBS and IC are multifactorial conditions with several proposed causes. Many of these causes may be altered during pregnancy, however, there is little published information about the changes in PBS/IC symptoms that may occur during pregnancy.

Of the commonly used oral PBS/IC treatments, pentosan polysulfate and amitriptyline have the lowest risks, and hydroxyzine has more risks.

Of the usual intravesical treatments, heparin is the safest because it is unlikely to be absorbed from the bladder or to cross the placenta. Intravesical lidocaine, as packaged, has minimal systemic absorption after intravesical administration. However, alkalinized lidocaine is absorbed from the bladder and gives serum levels approaching or within the therapeutic range. Lidocaine does cross the placenta and there is no information about the safety of chronic exposure to the fetus. DMSO and systemic corticosteroids have known teratogenic effects, but the absorption of intravesical corticosteroids is unknown.

Sacral nerve stimulators should not be placed during pregnancy and, if present already, should be turned off for the duration of pregnancy.

In a few cases, multiple members of the same family have IC. This suggests that some patients may have a genetic predisposition to develop IC. However, the vast majority of first-degree relatives of patients who have IC do not have the syndrome. Unless she belongs to a family that has multiple members with IC, the pregnant patient can be reassured that the risk for passing it on to her child is low.

References

[1] Abrams P, Cardozo L, Fall M, et al. The standardization of terminology in lower urinary tract function: report from the standardisation sub-committee of the International Continence Society. Neurourol Urodyn 2002;21(2):167–78.

[2] Teng J, Wang ZY, Bjorling DE. Estrogen-induced proliferation of urothelial cells is modulated by nerve growth factor. Am J Physiol Renal Physiol 2002;282(6):F1075–83.

[3] Teng J, Wang ZY, Bjorling DE. Progesterone induces the proliferation of urothelial cells in an epidermal growth factor dependent manner. J Urol 2003;170(5):2014–8.

[4] Wang XN, Das SK, Damm D, et al. Differential regulation of heparin-binding epidermal growth factor-like growth factor in the adult ovariectomized mouse uterus by progesterone and estrogen. Endocrinology 1994;135(3):1264–71.

[5] Okragly AJ, Niles AL, Saban R, et al. Elevated tryptase, nerve growth factor, neurotrophin-3 and glial cell line-derived neurotrophic factor levels in the urine of interstitial cystitis and bladder cancer patients. J Urol 1999;161(2):438–41.

[6] Lowe EM, Anand P, Terenghi G, et al. Increased nerve growth factor levels in the urinary bladder of women with idiopathic sensory urgency and interstitial cystitis. Br J Urol 1997;79(4):572–7.

[7] Keay SK, Zhang CO, Shoenfelt J, et al. Sensitivity and specificity of antiproliferative factor, heparin-binding epidermal growth factor-like growth factor, and epidermal growth factor as urine markers for interstitial cystitis. Urology 2001;57(6, Suppl 1):9–14.

[8] Theoharides TC, Pang X, Letourneau R, et al. Interstitial cystitis: a neuroimmunoendocrine disorder. Ann N Y Acad Sci 1998;840:619–34.

[9] Cutolo M, Sulli A, Capellino S, et al. Sex hormones influence on the immune system: basic and clinical aspects in autoimmunity. Lupus 2004;13(9):635–8.

[10] McEwen BS. Invited review: estrogen effects on the brain: multiple sites and molecular mechanisms. J Appl Physiol 2001;91(6):2785–801.

[11] Leonelli E, Ballabio M, Consoli A, et al. Neuroactive steroids: a therapeutic approach to maintain peripheral nerve integrity during neurodegenerative events. J Mol Neurosci 2006;28(1):65–76.

[12] Gintzler AR, Liu NJ. The maternal spinal cord: biochemical and physiological correlates of steroid-activated antinociceptive processes. Prog Brain Res 2001;133:83–97.

[13] Whitmore KE. Self-care regimens for patients with interstitial cystitis. Urol Clin North Am 1994;21(1):121–30.

[14] Simon LJ, Landis JR, Erickson DR, et al. The interstitial cystitis data base (ICDB): concepts and preliminary baseline descriptive statistics. Urology 1997;49(Suppl 5A):64–75.

[15] Onwude JL, Selo-Ojeme DO. Pregnancy outcomes following the diagnosis of interstitial cystitis. Gynecol Obstet Invest 2003;56(3):160–2.

[16] Andres RL. Effects of therapeutic, diagnostic and environmental agents and exposure to social and illicit drugs. In: Creasy RK, Resnik R, editors. Maternal fetal medicine: principles and practice. 5th edition. Philadelphia: WB Saunders; 2004. p. 281–314.

[17] Elmiron. In: Physicians' Desk Reference, 60th edition. Montvale (NJ): Thompson PDR; 2006. p. 2393–5.

[18] Erickson DR, Sheykhnazari M, Bhavanandan VP. Molecular size affects urine excretion of pentosanpolysulfate. J Urol 2006;175(3):1143–7.

[19] Amitriptyline. In: Briggs GG, Freeman RK, Yaffe SJ, editors. Drugs in pregnancy and lactation. 6th edition. Philadelphia: Lippincott, Williams & Wilkins; 2002. p. 59–62.

[20] Heikkinen T, Ekblad U, Laine K. Transplacental transferof amitriptyline and nortriptyline in isolated perfused human placenta. Psychopharm (Berlin) 2001;153(4):450–4.

[21] Elavil. In: Physicians' Desk Reference, 53rd edition. Montvale (NJ): Medical Economics Company; 1999. p. 3418–20.

[22] Wen SW, Walker M. Risk of fetal exposure to tricyclic antidepressants. J Obstet Gynaecol Can 2004;26(10):887–92.

[23] Eberhard-Gran M, Eskild A, Opjordsmoen S. Treating mood disorders during pregnancy: safety considerations. Drug Saf 2005;28(8):695–706.

[24] Nulman I, Rovet J, Stewart DE, et al. Child development following exposure to tricyclic antidepressants of fluoxetine throughout fetal life:

a prospective, controlled study. Am J Psych 2002; 159(11):1889–95.

[25] Nulman I, Rovet J, Stewart DE, et al. Neurodevelopment of children exposed in utero to antidepressant drugs. N Engl J Med 1997;336(4):258–62.

[26] Simon GE, Cunningham ML, Davis RL. Outcomes of prenatal antidepressant exposure. Am J Psych 2002;159(12):2055–61.

[27] Baldessarini RJ. Drugs and the treatment of psychiatric disorders: depression and anxiety disorders. In: Hardman JG, Limbird LE, editors. Goodman and Gilman's: The pharmacological basis of therapeutics. 10th edition. New York: McGraw-Hill; 2001. p. 447–83.

[28] Tetralogy. Drugs and other medications. In: Cunningham FG, Leveno KJ, Bloom SL, Houth JC, Gilstrap LC, Wenstrom KD, editors. Williams Obstetrics. 22nd edition. New York: McGraw-Hill; 2005. p. 341–71.

[29] van Ophoven A, Pokupic S, Heinecke A, et al. A prospective, randomized, placebo controlled, double-blind study of amitriptyline for the treatment of interstitial cystitis. J Urol 2004;172(2):533–6.

[30] Hydroxyzine. In: Briggs GG, Freeman RK, Yaffe SJ, editors. Drugs in pregnancy and lactation, 6th edition. Philadelphia: Lippincott, Williams & Wilkins; 2002. p. 679–82.

[31] Atarax. In: Physicians' Desk Reference, 53rd edition. Montvale (NJ): Medical Economics Company; 1999. p. 2367–8.

[32] Gilbert C, Mazzotta P, Loebstein R, et al. Fetal safety of drugs used in the treatment of allergic rhinitis: a critical review. Drug Saf 2005;28(8):707–19.

[33] Serreau R, Komiha M, Blanc F, et al. Neonatal seizures associated with maternal hydroxyzine hydrochloride in late pregnancy. Reprod Toxicol 2005; 20(4):573–4.

[34] Sant GR, Propert KJ, Hanno PM, et al. A pilot clinical trial of oral pentosan polysulfate and oral hydroxyzine in patients with interstitial cystitis. J Urol 2003;170(3):810–5.

[35] Zyrtec. In: Physicians' Desk Reference, 60th edition. Montvale (NJ): Thompson PDR; 2006. p. 2598–93.

[36] Einarson A, Bailey B, Jung G, et al. Prospective controlled study of hydroxyzine and cetirizine in pregnancy. Ann Allergy Asthma Immunol 1997;78(2): 183–6.

[37] Raffa RB. Antihistamines as analgesics. J Clin Pharm Ther 2001;26(2):81–5.

[38] Namazi MR. Cetirizine and allopurinol as novel weapons against cellular autoimmune disorders. Int Immunopharmacol 2004;4(3):349–53.

[39] Baroody FM, Naclerio RM. Antiallergic effects of H_1-receptor antagonists. Allergy 2000;55(Suppl 64): 117–27.

[40] Abdelaziz MM, Khair OA, Devalia JL. The potential of active metabolites of antihistamines in the management of allergic disease. Allergy 2000;55(5): 425–34.

[41] Rimso-50. In: Physicians' Desk Reference, 44th edition. Oradell (NJ): Medical Economics Company; 1990. p. 1743–4.

[42] Rozman KK, Klassen CD. Absorption, distribution and excretion of toxicants. In: Classed CD, editor. Casarett and Doull's toxicology. 6th edition. New York: McGraw-Hill; 2001. p. 107–32.

[43] Henry R, Patterson L, Avery N, et al. Absorption of alkalinized intravesical lidocaine in normal and inflamed bladders: a simple method for improving bladder anesthesia. J Urol 2001; 165(6):1900–3.

[44] Xylocaine. In: Physicians' Desk Reference, 53rd edition. Montvale (NJ): Medical Economics Company; 1999. p. 603–6.

[45] Amano T, Ohkawa M, Kunimi K, et al. Topical anesthesia for bladder biopsies and cautery: intravesical lidocaine versus caudal anesthesia. Int Urol Nephrol 1995;27(5):533–7.

[46] Asklin B, Cassuto J. Intravesical lidocaine in severe interstitial cystitis. Scand J Urol Nephrol 1989;23(4): 311–2.

[47] Clapp CR, Poss WB, Cilento BG. Lidocaine toxicity secondary to postoperative bladder instillation in a pediatric patient. Urology 1999;53(6):1228.

[48] Parsons CL. Successful downregulation of bladder sensory nerves with combination of heparin and alkalinized lidocaine in patients with interstitial cystitis. Urology 2005;65(1):454–8.

[49] Lidocaine. In: Briggs GG, Freeman RK, Yaffe SJ, editors. Drugs in pregnancy and lactation. 6th edition. Philadelphia: Lippincott, Williams & Wilkins; 2002. p. 788–90.

[50] Hydrocortisone. In: Briggs GG, Freeman RK, Yaffe SJ, editors. Drugs in pregnancy and lactation. 6th edition. Philadelphia: Lippincott, Williams & Wilkins; 2002. p. 662–70.

[51] Oren D, Nulman I, Makhija M, et al. Using corticosteroids during pregnancy. Are topical, inhaled, or systemic agents associated with risk? Can Fam Physician 2004;50:1083–5.

[52] Mattioli F, Tognoni P, Manfredi V, et al. Interindividual variability in the absorption of ciprofloxacin and hydrocortisone from continent ileal reservoir for urine. Eur J Clin Pharmacol 2006; 62(2):119–21.

[53] Roberts RO, Bergstralh EJ, Bass SE, et al. Incidence of physician-diagnosed interstitial cystitis in Olmsted County: a community-based study. BJU Int 2003;91(3):181–5.

[54] Curhan GC, Speizer FE, Hunter DJ, et al. Epidemiology of interstitial cystitis: a population based study. J Urol 1999;161(2):549–52.

[55] Clemens JQ, Meenan RT, Rosetti MC, et al. Prevalence and incidence of interstitial cystitis in a managed care population. J Urol 2005;173(1): 98–102.

[56] Clemens JQ, Meenan RT, O'Keeffe Rosetti MC, et al. Prevalence of interstitial cystitis symptoms in

a managed care population. J Urol 2005;174(2): 576–80.

[57] Rosenberg MT, Hazzard M. Prevalence of interstitial cystitis symptoms in women: a population based study in the primary care office. J Urol 2005;174(6): 2231–4.

[58] Parsons CL, Tatsis V. Prevalence of interstitial cystitis symptoms in young women. Urology 2004;64(5): 866–70.

[59] Warren JW, Jackson TL, Langenberg P, et al. Prevalence of interstitial cystitis in first-degree relatives of patients with interstitial cystitis. Urology 2004;63(1): 17–21.

[60] Koziol JA. Epidemiology of interstitial cystitis. Urol Clin North Am 1994;21(1):7–20.

[61] Warren JW, Keay SK, Meyers D, et al. Concordance of interstitial cystitis in monozygotic and dizygotic twin pairs. Urology 2001;57(Suppl 6A):22–5.

[62] Dimitrakov JD. A case of familial clustering of interstitial cystitis and chronic pelvic pain syndrome. Urology 2001;58(2):281.

[63] Dimitrakov JD, Boyden SE, Freeman MR, et al. Single nucleotide polymorphism (SNP) analysis of autosomal dominant interstitial cystitis: a family-based study. J Urol 2005;173(Suppl 4):84 [abstract 303].

ELSEVIER
SAUNDERS

Urol Clin N Am 34 (2007) 71–88

UROLOGIC
CLINICS
of North America

Pregnancy and Urinary Diversion

Richard E. Hautmann, MD*, Bjoern G. Volkmer, MD

Department of Urology, University of Ulm, Prittwitzstr 43, 89075 Ulm, Germany

In postmenopausal women, most urinary diversions are performed during oncologic surgery. In most children or premenopausal women who need urinary diversion, the underlying disease is benign. Among these are complex malformations (eg, bladder exstrophy), neurogenic bladder, or contracted bladders after tuberculosis or interstitial cystitis.

After the problems associated with urinary incontinence have been resolved, and the patients have reached puberty, sexuality and fertility become more significant. At this time, the medical responsibility shifts from the pediatrician and pediatric urologist to the gynecologist and general practitioner. These clinicians rarely have major experience, however, with the psychological aspects of sexuality, fertility, and pregnancy in these patients [1]. All functions of female sexuality can be preserved if a fertility-sparing cystectomy and urinary diversion—including a neobladder—are performed [2]. Consequently, the patient's desire for a normal sexual life has to be respected.

These patients pose a dilemma because they present with two rare conditions: They have a disease that has led to deterioration of their bladder function, and their urinary tract was diverted by extended reconstructive procedures. The underlying disease and urinary diversion are accompanied by specific problems. Depending on the underlying disease, difficulties with conception and pregnancy continue to be a problem despite the availability of in vitro fertilization and careful obstetric care [3]. Many

women with urinary diversion come to pregnancy with an attitude of some determination. They realize the possibility of there being problems and likely are prepared to face these [4]. A woman with a urinary diversion who becomes pregnant soon realizes that her case is a unique constellation—not comparable to any other pregnancy. In women with urinary diversion, there are numerous influencing factors (eg, age, underlying disease, genetic implications, pelvic anatomy, concomitant abnormalities, intra-abdominal adhesions, renal function, form of urinary diversion, presentation of the fetus, infections of the urinary tract). In this situation, women with urinary diversions do not have the opportunity to discuss issues related to pregnancy, labor, and delivery with other women who have had this experience. Their obstetricians may not have experience with patients with a comparable condition. In a questionnaire survey, women stated that they had felt alone as they faced pregnancy with urinary diversion or ostomy [5].

The first case of pregnancy in a woman with a ureterosigmoidostomy was reported in 1922 by Knauf [6]. Since then, only 252 cases of pregnancy after urinary diversion have been published in the literature. A survey in 1965 revealed that only 1 in 10,000 obstetric admissions in major medical centers was related to pregnancy in patients with urinary diversion [7]. Despite growing experience with urinary diversion, only a limited number of patients are suitable for a fertility-sparing approach. Optimized treatment options helped many patients, who were candidates for urinary diversion in the past, to avoid this operation today.

Every woman with a urinary diversion has become an expert regarding her body and its

---

* Corresponding author.

E-mail address: richard.hautmann@uniklinik-ulm.de (R.E. Hautmann).

functions and wishes to be as involved as possible in all decisions and in her own care. These women already have undergone major surgical procedures, leaving numerous abdominal and pubic scars that they regard as a severe detriment to their appearance. Most have an ostomy that requires the constant wearing of a bag-type appliance, and by the time they have reached their marriage age, they may be close to the limit for tolerating medical problems and hospitalizations. They may have insecurities as to their desirability to their husbands and would not want to risk any other problems that a pregnancy might cause in this regard. Guidance should be given to these women by their physicians, making clear to them the possible complications and side effects of childbearing [8].

In the authors' center, with a large expertise in urinary diversion, the number of cases with pregnancies is limited. The authors have observed four women with a total of five successful pregnancies. Three women had a ureterosigmoidostomy and one had an ileal neobladder—the only case published to date. The authors also performed a literature review, which revealed a total of 188 women who altogether had 252 pregnancies. There were 222 children alive and doing well, 7 pregnancy terminations, 14 abortions, and 9 stillbirths. This article uses this prior experience to provide guidance for urologists, obstetricians, general practitioners, and patients to aid decision making in pregnancies after urinary diversion.

General physiologic changes during pregnancy

General physiologic changes that are encountered during pregnancy are listed in Table 1 [9–13]. Changes of the upper and lower urinary tracts also are discussed in other articles in this issue.

Special urologic problems during pregnancy in patients with urinary diversion using bowel segments

The population of women with pregnancy after urinary diversion is extremely inhomogeneous. Some women had cystectomy, and others did not. Cystectomy is inevitable before creating an ileal neobladder, but in all other forms of urinary diversion, it is not mandatory, as long as no malignant disease of the urinary bladder

is present. (With bladder exstrophy, techniques for bladder reconstruction have evolved only more recently, so most patients of childbearing years with bladder exstrophy have undergone cystectomy.) In patients with cystectomy, the pelvic floor may have reduced elasticity as a result of scarring. If the peritoneum was entered during the cystectomy, the patient may have severe adhesions of the intestine at the ventral abdominal wall and in the true pelvis that might be relevant during the enlargement of the uterus in pregnancy and in case of a cesarean section.

Any operation for urinary diversion should fulfill two general criteria: It should be clinically acceptable for the surgeon, and it should be socially and psychologically acceptable for the patient [14]. Since the early twentieth century, there have been significant changes in the techniques of urinary diversion, with the goal to improve patients' quality of life. Among these considerations, pregnancy played a minor role because it was relevant for only a few women with urinary diversion. Pregnancies that occur after urinary tract reconstruction can have a significant effect on function of the reconstructed urinary tract, and the reconstruction can significantly affect the delivery of the fetus [15]. Also, urinary diversion with or without cystectomy may lead to problems that become overt only during pregnancy. There is no recommendation as yet for what type of urinary diversion should be chosen in girls or women who might want to become pregnant. Analyzing the previous literature, the authors found no case in which a certain form of urinary diversion was preferred with respect to a planned pregnancy.

Fixation of the uterus

Any surgical manipulation to the true pelvis or to the intestine may lead to visceral adhesions. Especially in patients with rectal surgery, a tendency toward uterine retroflexion was observed [16]. This tendency may negatively influence fertility because of difficulties in conception and in implantation of the blastocyst. The enlargement of the uterus during pregnancy may cause intestinal obstruction and ileus.

Fixation of the bowel segment

The bowel segments used for urinary diversion have at least three fixation points: the site of

Table 1
Physiologic changes of pregnancy

	First trimester	Second trimester	Third trimester
Blood	Blood volume ↑ Plasma volume ↑ RBC ↑	Blood volume ↑ Plasma volume ↑↑ RBC ↑ **Hemodilution**	Blood volume 25–40% ↑ Plasma volume 50% ↑ RBC 15% ↑ **Hemodilution**
Cardiovascular system		Cardiac output ↑ Systemic vascular resistance ↓	Cardiac output 30–50% ↑ Systemic vascular resistance ↓ Compression of the great vessels
Respiratory system		FRC ↓ Oxygen consumption ↑	FRC 20% ↓ Oxygen consumption 15% ↑ **Risk of hypoxemia during hypoventilation ↑**
Coagulation system		Factor VII, VIII, X ↑ Fibrinogen ↑ Fibrinolysis ↓ Velocity of venous blood flow (lower extremity) ↑ Venous pressure ↑ **Risk of venous thromboembolism ↑**	Factor VII, VIII, X ↑ Fibrinogen ↑ Fibrinolysis ↓ Velocity of venous blood flow (lower extremity) ↑ Venous pressure ↑ **Risk of venous thromboembolism ↑↑**
Gastrointestinal tract	Gastric motility ↓ Gastroesophageal sphincter activity ↓ Gastric pH ↓ Time of gastrointestinal transit ↑	Gastric motility ↓ Gastroesophageal sphincter activity ↓ Gastric pH ↓ Intra-abdominal pressure ↑ **Gastroesophageal reflux, aspiration ↑** Time of gastrointestinal transit ↑	Gastric motility ↓ Gastroesophageal sphincter activity ↓ Gastric pH ↓ Intra-abdominal pressure ↑ **Gastroesophageal reflux, aspiration ↑↑** Time of gastrointestinal transit ↑
Urinary tract	Dilated upper urinary tract (R > L) (↑) Relative urinary stasis GFR ↑ Serum creatinine ↓ Blood urea nitrogen ↓ Bladder = extraperitoneal	Dilated upper urinary tract (R > L) ↑ Relative urinary stasis GFR ↑ Serum creatinine ↓ Blood urea nitrogen ↓ Bladder = extraperitoneal	Dilated upper urinary tract (R > L) ↑ Relative urinary stasis GFR ↑ Serum creatinine ↓ Blood urea nitrogen ↓ Bladder = intraperitoneal

Abbreviations: FRC, functional residual capacity; GFR, glomerular filtration rate; RBC, red blood cell count.
Data from references [9–13].

ureteral implantation, the mesentery, and the site of the efferent segment (eg, the ostomy in conduits or pouches or the anastomosis to the urethra or the trigone in neobladders or augmentation enterocystoplasties). In ureterosigmoidostomies, these three fixation points are fused to one single fixation at the ureterosigmoidal anastomosis. Intra-abdominal changes during pregnancy may lead to a separation of these fixation points. The stoma will be located in a more and more lateral position. This may lead to stretching of the bowel segment. For the long-term functioning of the urinary diversion, the reversibility of such processes is crucial because permanent enlargement of the bowel segment may lead to incomplete emptying and residual urine after delivery.

Compression of the ureter and the bowel segment by the uterus

In patients with an intact urinary tract, the urinary bladder usually is compressed between the enlarging uterus and the abdominal wall and the symphysis, whereas the ureters may be entrapped between the uterus and the bony pelvic ring. Because pouches, neobladders, and enterocystoplasties are located ventrally to the uterus, a compression by the uterus inevitably occurs, worsening the storage function of the reservoir. The risk of ureteral compression depends mainly on the length of the ureters (inside/outside the true pelvis), on the transposition of the ureter to the contralateral side, and on the implantation technique.

Perfusion of the bowel segment

Especially in diversions with fixation to the pelvic floor or abdominal wall, the growing uterus may lead to a chronic tension of the mesentery and blood supply to the bowel segment. The potential effect is largest in patients with neobladders or enterocystoplasties. An acute tension of the mesentery may decrease perfusion of the reservoir. A slowly increasing tension of the mesentery during pregnancy leaves enough time for adaptation of the blood supply.

Intestinal obstruction

In two early reports of patients with urinary or intestinal diversion, the incidence of intestinal obstruction during pregnancy was 10% [17,18]. In the authors' analysis of the 252 published cases, however, they found no case with a significant intestinal obstruction after urinary diversion. The authors concluded that this complication may be limited to ostomates with intestinal diseases. These patients usually have undergone several intestinal manipulations, leading to an increased risk of intestinal adhesions and obstruction.

Stenosis and prolapse of the urostomy

In patients with continent or wet urostomy, the growing intra-abdominal pressure during pregnancy may lead to parastomal hernia or stomal prolapse. Compression of the efferent limb of the pouch or conduit may affect a stenosis of the stoma. These problems may be transient or permanent. Several cases with a stoma repair during cesarean section have been reported.

Metabolic complications

The absence of large portions of intestine may give rise to malabsorption states. In pregnancy, these may become more significant. Thought must be given to folic acid and vitamin B_{12} supplements. The disturbance of bowel function caused by oral iron supplements may be a real nuisance to patients with urinary diversion, and parenteral iron may become necessary [19]. Electrolyte imbalance in women with urinary diversion is much more likely to occur than in other women. This imbalance may be as a result of hyperemesis or may occur in labor. Despite the fact that pregnancy is essentially a hypercalciuric state, the incidence of stone formation is not increased because of several physiologic factors that mitigate against stone formation. Calcium stone inhibitors, such as citrate and magnesium, are excreted in the urine in increased amounts during pregnancy [20].

Renal function in the course of pregnancy

In many women with malformations of the urinary tract or neurogenic bladders, impaired renal function is the main indication for urinary diversion. At least 11 of 188 patients (6%) with pregnancy after urinary diversion had a history of unilateral nephrectomy. The type of diversion depends on the renal function. Cutaneous ureterostomies or conduits are indicated even in patients with severely impaired renal function. Pouches, neobladders, and ureterosigmoidostomies are limited to patients with good or slightly impaired renal function (generally serum creatinine <2 mg/dL) because the resorption in the intestinal segments and the metabolic imbalance put a heavy strain on the excretory capacity of the kidneys. Mild renal tract dilation is a common finding during pregnancy. Renal tract dilation tends to occur after the seventh week and is more prominent to the right side. In women with urinary diversion, urinary tract infections and hydronephrosis are expected to occur more frequently [21]. Any abnormal renal function is aggravated by the pregnancy, altering the prognosis [22]. At least one case of fatal postpartum renal failure has been reported [23].

Impact of the underlying disease on the urinary diversion

In the authors' review to 2005, 188 patients with urinary diversion became pregnant. As shown in Table 2, most patients had bladder

Table 2
Women ($N = 188$) with pregnancy after urinary diversion: underlying disease and form of urinary diversion

	Ureterosigmoidostomy	Ileal conduit	Colonic conduit	Continent pouch	Enterocystoplasty	Neobladder	Total
Bladder exstrophy	47	18	1	10	5	0	81
Myelomeningocele	0	19	0	2	6	0	27
Neurogenic bladder	0	13	0	3	11	1	28
Interstitial/chronic cystitis	4	2	0	0	6	0	12
Tuberculous contracted bladder	2	0	0	0	10	0	12
Complex fistula	1	0	0	1	2	0	4
Complex malformations	1	2	0	2	1	0	6
Malignant tumor	1	0	0	1	0	0	2
Miscellaneous/ unknown	8	2	0	0	6	0	16
Total	64	56	1	19	47	1	188

exstrophy or neurogenic bladders of varying origin (eg, trauma, myelomeningocele, unknown). Ureterosigmoidostomy was chosen mainly in exstrophy cases. Continent urinary diversion to the urethra (enterocystoplasty or neobladder) was mainly restricted to cases with low-capacity contracted bladders (eg, neurogenic bladder, interstitial cystitis, tuberculous cystitis). Most patients with myelomeningocele received ileal conduits.

Bladder exstrophy

Bladder exstrophy is a congenital anomaly characterized by absence of the anterior bladder wall, eversion of the posterior bladder wall, and other abnormalities. The urethra is usually absent; cleft or absent clitoris, wide labial separation with exposure of the vaginal orifice, defect of the anterior vaginal wall, wide separation of the symphysis pubis, and anomalies of the vagina and uterus are frequent [24]. Infants today with classic bladder exstrophy can expect a normal life span. Although sexual activity in a young woman with bladder exstrophy is common, it is not universal. In a study by Burbige and colleagues [3], only 8 of the 12 patients surveyed (19–33 years old) were sexually active; 6 of the 8 patients reported regular orgasm, and 4 reported significant dyspareunia, which did not seem to be related to age or obstetric history. Five of six

patients who desired pregnancy became pregnant. Pregnancy in a woman with bladder exstrophy was first reported in 1724 by Bonnet [25].

Genetic counseling

In current estimates, the risk of transmission of bladder exstrophy to progeny is about 1 in 70 to 1 in 100. Based on these findings, occurrence of bladder exstrophy seems to be multifactorial rather than directly genetically based; combined environmental and developmental factors may play a significant role in the cause of the exstrophy-epispadias complex [26]. In our complete series of 252 pregnancies, complex malformations (anencephalus, myelomeningocele, stillbirth) were observed in only one child, whose mother had myelomeningocele and bladder exstrophy. This mother had another pregnancy with a healthy child several years later [27].

Malformations of the external and internal genitalia

Reconstruction of the external genitalia, with adaptation of the bifid clitoris and divergent mons pubis, usually shows satisfactory cosmetic results. Nevertheless, in some cases, multiple operations for bladder reconstruction can result in ugly scars on the abdominal wall, whereas in others the mons pubis may remain split medially and divided by a huge hairless scar [1]. Also, women with bladder exstrophy usually have a narrow vaginal introitus. This can be corrected by episiotomy or vaginoplasty. The definitive introitoplasty should be performed before cohabitation. At the time of definitive cutback, antefixation of the uterus is recommended because otherwise uterine prolapse of several degrees may occur [1].

Uterine malformations were found in 7 of 81 patients who became pregnant after urinary diversion for bladder exstrophy: 5 had a bicornuate uterus, and 2 had a uterus didelphys. Only one of these patients had an abortion. Even these severe malformations do not impair the fertility of the affected women. When pregnancy is achieved, however, uterine prolapse may be a problem, owing to the lack of pelvic floor support structures [28].

Malpresentation

Patients with bladder exstrophy had a 25% incidence of abnormal fetal presentation, leading to a higher risk for cesarean section [25]. Malpresentation of the fetus is probably due to the widely split pelvis, which fails to control the presenting part [8].

Prolapse of the cervix or uterus

Pelvic organ prolapse is a complex disorder that potentially involves not only poor support for multiple sites in the vagina, but also the function of the urethra, bladder, and anorectum and sexual function [29]. Bladder outflow obstruction as a result of severe cervical prolapse should be treated with bed rest and indwelling catheter placement if clean intermittent catheterization is impaired [30].

Vaginal delivery may aggravate an underlying tendency to genital prolapse [31]. Clemetson [25] recommended that if prolapse occurs before labor, vaginal delivery should be encouraged. He suggested that if prolapse does not occur antepartum, a cesarean section is necessary to prevent prolapse developing later. Prolapse of the cervix or the uterus was present to various extents during 33 of 122 pregnancies in patients with bladder exstrophy (27%). One third of these patients had a vaginal delivery, and two thirds had a cesarean section. One patient had four pregnancies with three cesarean sections, despite recurring cervical prolapse [32]. In total, only five patients had any form of parametrial fixation during follow-up.

Neurogenic bladder

General problems
Pathophysiology of uterine contractions. Depending on the level of the neurologic lesion, patients with spinal cord injury or spina bifida may not detect the onset of labor, especially preterm labor [33]. Paraplegia does not affect the ability of the uterus to contract normally [34], but may preclude the coordinated muscle effort necessary for the final stages of labor [31,33]. These factors may necessitate cesarean delivery to protect the urinary reconstruction, especially if prolonged or difficult labor is anticipated.

Motility of the lower limbs. Fixed adduction deformity at the hips, with inability to abduct the thighs adequately, also has been reported as an indication for cesarean section [35,36].

Fecal incontinence. Fecal incontinence may be a problem in all patients with ureterosigmoidostomy. Combined urinary and fecal incontinence leads to a significant reduction of the quality of life. Before choosing this type of urinary diversion, verification of an intact rectal sphincter is mandatory. Fecal incontinence also presents a problem in all patients with urinary diversion to the urethra (eg, neobladders), to the perineum, or to the lower abdomen. Because these patients usually wear diapers, the risk of contamination of the urethral orifice or the stoma with bacteria from the intestine and the risk of urinary tract infections are high.

Problems specific to meningomyelocele
Genetic counseling. Neural tube defect is regarded as a multifactorial disorder in which multiple genetic factors and environmental factors may play a role. The risk of neural tube defect in offspring of spina bifida parents was 4.1% (11 of 267 children) [37].

Anatomic changes of the bony pelvis. Patients with spina bifida have varying degrees of muscular weakness, which, over the years, may result in secondary skeletal abnormalities. The effects of muscular paralysis on the pelvis are pelvic asymmetry and lumbosacral scoliosis [33,38]. A patient with spina bifida is likely to have an abnormal pelvis, which could make a vaginal delivery difficult or impossible. Abnormal pelvic dimensions can result in abnormal presentation of the fetus, such as breech or persistent parietal presentation [39]. Careful assessment of the pelvis is necessary. In patients with a poorly developed sacrum, the pelvic cavity may be surprisingly spacious. Wynn and coworkers [40] stated that if the head is capable of engaging normally in the pelvis, vaginal delivery should be successfully achieved. When pelvic assessment shows reduced measurements, a cesarean section should be planned.

One hazardous effect that pregnancy may have in a paraplegic patient is increased abdominal pressure on the paralyzed diaphragm. This pressure may result from increasing uterine size and marked distention of the large intestine caused by fecal impaction, and it may increase any hypoxia.

Additional malformations. Neural tube defects are associated with congenital or functional urinary tract abnormalities. The most common congenital malformation is unilateral renal agenesis. Also, abnormalities in fusion or migration of renal tissue are common, resulting in renal abnormalities, such as a horseshoe kidney, pelvic kidney, or crossed ectopia. Occurring less commonly, although more frequently than in the general population, are congenital abnormalities of the lower urinary tract [41]. A high incidence of latex allergy also has been reported in these patients [42,43].

Ventriculoperitoneal shunt. Hydrocephalus develops in 65% to 85% of patients with myelomeningocele, and 5% to 10% of myelomeningocele patients have clinically overt hydrocephalus at birth [44]. More than 80% of patients with myelomeningocele who develop hydrocephalus do so before age 6 months. Most patients have an associated Chiari type 2 malformation [45]. Ventriculoperitoneal shunts are the most common cerebrospinal fluid shunts used in hydrocephalus patients today. Shunt malfunction may occur in pregnancy. These patients present with headache, with nausea and vomiting, with or without gaze palsy, and sometimes with impaired consciousness [37]. These symptoms may mimic preeclampsia, which must be ruled out [46]. The enlarging uterus, possibly through the impedance of cerebrospinal fluid flow through the shunt owing to relatively increased intra-abdominal pressure, is largely responsible for the symptoms of shunt obstruction [47,48]. Another possibility is that the peritoneal catheter becomes compressed between the uterus and other viscera [47].

Vaginal delivery in patients with a ventriculoperitoneal shunt is preferable, and cesarean section should be performed only for obstetric reasons [49,50]. Opening the peritoneal cavity at cesarean section carries the risk of septicemic infection of the cerebrospinal fluid shunt. Kleinman and colleagues [51] recommended an extraperitoneal approach at cesarean section to protect the shunt from infection.

Trauma

Trauma leading to a neurogenic bladder has been reported in only one case with pregnancy after urinary diversion [52].

Miscellaneous

There were only two reports on patients who had radical cystectomy and urinary diversion for malignant tumors. One patient had a bladder rhabdomyosarcoma. After radical cystectomy and formation of an Indiana pouch, she successfully became pregnant three times. Repeat elective cesarean sections were performed without any damage to the reservoir [53]. The other patient had urachal carcinoma. Two years after radical cystectomy and ureterosigmoidostomy, she delivered a healthy child vaginally. She died from tumor progression 2 years later [54]. These cases show that patients with malignant diseases may be at a lifelong risk of tumor recurrence.

Special problems during pregnancy depending on the type of urinary diversion

Ureterosigmoidostomy

Ureterosigmoidostomy was the first continent urinary diversion. It provided a normal body image with perfect social integration and normal sexual behavior in the long-term course [1,55]. The longest reported follow-up with ureterosigmoidostomy was 59 years [56]. Fecal continence and an intact anal sphincter are the prerequisites for this form of urinary diversion.

Upper urinary tract infections

Although the ureter is implanted with antirefluxing techniques, the risk of bacterial ascension and upper urinary tract infections is still increased. Pyelonephritis is associated with a significant rate of fetal wastage, preterm birth, and small-for-dates infants [54,57]. Among 95 pregnancies in patients with ureterosigmoidostomy [6–8,22,23,32,54,56,58–93], 17 cases with feverish upper urinary tract infections were observed (18%). Two of these infections led to abortion. The rate of urinary tract infections did not differ significantly from the risk in the other types of urinary diversion, which was 16%.

Hydronephrosis

Hydronephrosis was observed during five pregnancies after ureterosigmoidostomy. This rate is distinctly lower than during normal pregnancies. This rate may depend on the localization of the ureterosigmoidal anastomosis. Because this anastomosis is usually located outside the true pelvis, the entrapment of the ureters between the growing uterus and the pelvic bone may be avoided. It has to be considered, however, that ultrasound was not yet available in most cases. Using ultrasound, the authors more recently diagnosed hydronephrosis in all four cases of a small contemporary series of pregnancies after ureterosigmoidostomy. The authors think that the rate of hydronephrosis and dilation of the upper urinary tract is underestimated in the literature. In differentiating acute obstruction of the upper urinary tract from chronic dilation, the resistive index proved to be a helpful tool [91]. In acute obstruction, hemodynamic changes reduce the diastolic flow and increase the resistive index greater than 0.7 [94].

Metabolic problems

The risk of long-term metabolic complications of ureterosigmoidostomy was unknown when most cases with pregnancy were reported. Many patients with urinary diversion to the colon develop some degree of azotemia and hyperchloremic acidosis caused by the intestinal reabsorption of chloride and ammonia, often combined with potassium loss [95]. Using substitution with sodium-potassium-hydrogencitrate when the base excess decreased to less than −2.5, no relevant imbalances could be observed in the authors' patients [91].

Damage to the anal sphincter

For a patient with ureterosigmoidostomy, an intact anal sphincter is crucial. Vaginal delivery may lead to injury to the rectum or anal sphincter. Lateral episiotomies are strongly recommended when vaginal delivery is chosen. With this regimen, there are no reports of rectal lacerations or postpartum anal incontinence [91].

Conduits

Ileal or colonic conduit is the most frequently used incontinent type of urinary diversion. Since 1969, 78 pregnancies were reported in patients with ileal conduits [1,3–5,8,27,33,35,52,54,95–110]. Most patients had myelomeningocele or other forms of neurogenic bladders. This type of diversion is even feasible in patients with reduced renal function, in patients with reduced dexterity to perform self-catheterization, and in patients with complex anomalies of the abdominal and pelvic anatomy, which would not allow some types of continent diversion.

Achieving continence may be challenging to the surgeon, but patients' experience with this condition is completely different. Eleven of 12 patients with an ileal conduit considered themselves to be continent, with 9 of 12 satisfied with the current situation [101].

Urinary tract infections

As in ureterosigmoidostomies, not all patients with urinary diversion previously underwent cystectomy. In patients with conduit diversions, the defunctionalized native bladder is occasionally the source of recurrent infections and pyocystis. Most of these respond, however, to bladder irrigation and antibiotics [17,111]. The risk of ascending urinary tract infections in ileal conduits is low. Risk factors during pregnancy are hydronephrosis and obstruction of the conduit.

Hydronephrosis

Transposition of the ureter within the retroperitoneal space to facilitate its anastomosis to the conduit might predispose to ureteral compression between the spine and the growing uterus [105]. Only three cases of hydronephrosis during pregnancy were reported, however.

Compression of the conduit

The effects of the enlarging uterus depend on how the ileal segment is situated in the abdomen. If the segment is retroperitoneal, the uterus can enlarge over it and may compress the segment to some extent. If the ileal segment is intraperitoneal and only loosely attached to the retroperitoneum and cecum, the enlarging uterus stretches the segment. This stretching is not always harmful, and after the delivery the loop may return to reasonable length. If not, it may be necessary to revise the ileostomy stoma by removing some length of ileal segment [7]. Stretching may be a more serious concern than compression, and it is recommended that the surgeon be certain to extraperitonealize the loop in female patients [70]. Only two cases of ileal conduit obstruction have been published [33,108]; this shows that most of the considerations made before are academic.

Problems of the stoma

Changes of the peristomal skin are common to all patients with urostomies. Early hormonal changes of pregnancy also can affect the peristomal skin. This is often first noticed by an ostomate when appliances do not stick well or need more frequent changing [4]. Also, as the abdomen enlarges, the stoma itself changes shape, often becoming more oval. It is vital to maintain an accurate fitting of the appliance, to avoid damage to the skin and stoma [4].

Leaks can occur when lying down because of the relative change in position of the stoma. As the abdomen enlarges, the stoma moves more lateral. This movement not only makes for difficulties in seeing the stoma when changing an appliance, but also for sleeping [4]. Cass and colleagues [98] reported on a case of severe ulceration of the stoma during pregnancy, which was fully reversible. Greenberg and associates [103] published one case with a stenosis of the stoma in the third trimester that required the insertion of a catheter. A prolapse of an ileal conduit was observed in only one case [8]. This patient had a vaginal delivery. Because the prolapse was not reversible, it had to be revised surgically. Postpartum, appliances need to be changed every couple of days, as the stoma and abdomen regain their former contours [4].

Pouches

The first pregnancy in a patient with a continent pouch in the technique described by Makkas [112] was reported by Forshell [113]. This patient with bladder exstrophy had an implantation of the trigone to the isolated cecum with an appendicocutaneostomy in 1917. The patient performed intermittent catheterization every 6 hours. Because a prolapse of the anterior vaginal wall was observed, a cesarean section was performed at 38 weeks of gestation to prevent further prolapse of the uterus. Six years later, the patient had cystitis-like symptoms. Radiologic examinations revealed a pouch filled with 13 concrements. A poucholithotomy was performed removing almost 200 g of stones.

Different types of pouches have since been developed. They vary in the intestinal segments and techniques used to construct the afferent segment, the reservoir, and the efferent segment. Since 1991, pregnancies have been reported in patients with Kock pouch, Indiana pouch, and Mainz pouch I [14,15,21,53,90,107,113–118]. Vaginal deliveries were possible with continent ileostomies [21], although the rate of vaginal delivery was only 27%.

Hydronephrosis

Seven of 26 patients (27%) developed hydronephrosis during pregnancy. If there is a compromise of renal function, premature labor, or severe cervical prolapse impeding clean intermittent catheterization, emergent or semielective cesarean section is recommended.

Urinary tract infections

Feverish urinary tract infections were observed only in patients with hydronephrosis. Five of 7 patients with hydronephrosis had urinary tract infections, whereas none of 19 patients without hydronephrosis were affected.

Catheterization

Patients who had the most difficulty were patients with a continent urinary diversion using an orthotopic Indiana pouch with a catheterizable ileal stoma in the perineum. In these patients, the catheterizable tube routinely elongated and became difficult to catheterize. Three of the five patients with this form of continent urinary diversion had to have an indwelling catheter in the third trimester [15].

Problems of the efferent segment

Hatch and colleagues [114] described a woman with an ileocecal pouch urinary reservoir who became increasingly incontinent in the third trimester and underwent cesarean section for breech presentation. Incontinence of the pouch was probably secondary to the increased intra-abdominal pressure on the reservoir from the gravid uterus.

Problems of the stoma

In one patient with a continent ileal reservoir, the continence nipple valve everted and prolapsed through the stoma. The patient herself manually reset the valve prolapse and voided more frequently. The function of the continence valve was normal postpartum [14].

Augmentation cystoplasty

Augmentation cystoplasty is a form of urinary diversion limited to patients with an intact sphincter. Most of these patients had contracted bladders. The most frequent etiologies were tuberculosis, schistosomiasis, interstitial cystitis, radiotherapy, repeat bladder operations, and neurogenic diseases of the bladder [119]. In 1889, von Mikulicz performed the first augmentation cystoplasty in a patient with bladder exstrophy [120]. This technique was popularized by Couvelaire in the 1950s [121]. Modern pharmacotherapy and clean intermittent self-catheterization have reduced the indications for this form of urinary diversion.

Different intestinal segments have been used for enterocystoplasty, including ileal, ileocecal, cecal, sigmoid, and gastric [119,122,123]. There are reports on pregnancies in 28 cases with ileal cystoplasty, 7 cases with ileocecal cystoplasty, 1 case with ileosigmoid cystoplasty, and 10 cases with colonic cystoplasty [15,36,90,102,124–143]. The average rate of clean intermittent self-catheterization after enterocystoplasty was 54% (range 14–100%) [119]. In a large contemporary series, 87% of patients with enterocystoplasty reported to be completely continent [144]. Some degree of sphincteric weakness seems to render the patient less prone to voiding difficulty after augmentation [144].

In selected patients with appropriate urinary tract function, bladder augmentation has made reproduction a more desirable option because of the improved physical appearance and self-image [129]. Especially in patients with a wet stoma, this may trigger the decision to undivert it to a colocystoplasty, as in two cases described by Bruce and coworkers [124]. One of these patients had two normal pregnancies postoperatively.

The first pregnancy in a patient with ureteroileocystoplasty for tuberculous cystitis was published in 1955 [130]. The altered urinary tract anatomy in patients with bladder augmentations may lead to antepartum and intrapartum complications. The mesenteric blood supply to the bladder augmentation potentially could be compromised by the enlarging uterus and lead to ischemia and hemorrhage. There are no reports, however, on disturbed perfusion of the intestinal segment used for augmentation during the course of pregnancy. Marked adhesions from previous extensive abdominopelvic surgeries and the position of the mesenteric blood supply of the bladder augmentation warrant special consideration in the event of amniocentesis or cesarean section (Figs. 1 and 2) [129]. In contrast to urinary diversions with a continent or a wet stoma in which the mesenteric pedicle of the intestinal segment extends cranially and laterally from the uterus, the mesenteric pedicle covers the uterus when there is an ileal substitute bladder [140].

The enterocystoplasty is entrapped by the enlarging uterus because it is fixed cranially by the mesentery, laterally by the ureters, and caudally by the trigone and urethra. During pregnancy, the mesentery elongates and is located

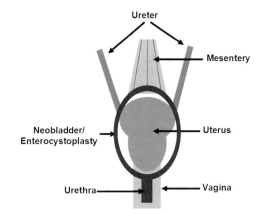

Fig. 1. Anatomic situs with enterocystoplasty or neobladder before pregnancy. The enterocystoplasty or neobladder is located ventrally to the uterus. Fixation points are the ureterointestinal anastomoses, the mesentery of the intestinal segment, and the trigone or urethra.

more and more laterally, and the uterus reaches the ventral abdominal wall. During cesarean section, there is a theoretical risk of damaging the augmentation or its mesentery. Among 16 published cases of cesarean section in patients with enterocystoplasty, however, no damage of the ileal segment or its blood supply was observed. Hill and colleagues [133] reported that the pedicle was simply pushed to one side of the uterus. Smith [145] described an ileal augmentation being pushed to the left side of the pelvis while the uterus was to right side. Most problems are thought to be avoided by performing a classic upper-segment section, rather than a lower-

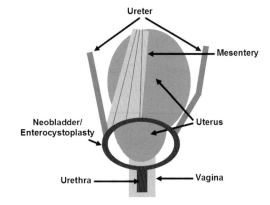

Fig. 2. Anatomic situs with enterocystoplasty or neobladder during pregnancy. The mesentery of the intestinal segment is elongated and placed more laterally, and the enlarged uterus reaches the ventral abdominal wall.

segment section [119]. The anatomic changes during pregnancy allow a secure approach to the upper ventral surface of the uterus.

Urinary tract infections

Asymptomatic bacteriuria occurs in 50% to 100% of patients with augmentation cystoplasty, but only 4% to 43% have significant urinary tract infections [146]. Among all pregnancies with augmentation cystoplasty, the rate of severe urinary tract infections during pregnancy was 17.4%. The risk of upper urinary tract infections depends on the presence of vesicoureteral reflux and on the necessity of self-catheterization. Especially in patients with reflux, long-term antibiotic prophylaxis during pregnancy may be indicated.

Hydronephrosis

Hydronephrosis during pregnancy was reported in only 2 of 46 cases. This low incidence is unexpected because, if augmentation cystoplasty is the only procedure, the ureters are untouched and cross the pelvic brim the same way in a normal pregnant woman. A possible explanation is that many of these reports are from an early time, when prenatal ultrasound was not used routinely.

Emptying of the bladder and catheterization

Half of patients with enterocystoplasty required clean intermittent self-catheterization before pregnancy—especially in cases with neurogenic bladders. During pregnancy, all patients in the series presented by Hensle and associates [15] had residual urine and required catheterization.

Continence

During pregnancy, 8 of 46 patients with enterocystoplasty had a new-onset stress urinary incontinence. In at least two cases, a permanent transurethral catheter was inserted at the 10 to 12 weeks of gestation.

There is some fear that vaginal delivery might damage the continence mechanism. Patients with a normal continence mechanism may be allowed to deliver vaginally, if there are no other obstetric contraindications. Patients who have undergone an augmentation cystoplasty and either vesical neck reconstruction or placement of an artificial genitourinary sphincter should undergo cesarean section, however, to avoid the potential for disruption of the continence mechanism [134]. There is only one report on a patient with an additional artificial sphincter. Cesarean section was uneventful in this case [134]. In one patient with a subtotal cystectomy and ileal substitute bladder

for interstitial cystitis, vaginal delivery with vacuum extraction led to urinary and fecal incontinence as a manifestation of a serious destabilization of the pelvic diaphragm [140]. There are reports on 26 uneventful vaginal deliveries without any impairment of the continence mechanism. Creagh and associates [147] recommended vaginal delivery as safe in patients with enterocystoplasty.

Metabolic complications

Metabolic consequences of cystoplasty are well known. Hyperchloremic acidosis, hypokalemia, hypocalcemia, hypomagnesemia, hyperammonemia, vitamin B_{12} deficiency, and steatorrhea are more or less frequent according to the intestinal segment incorporated in bladder augmentation [148]. In a series with long-term follow-up, however, the overall rate of metabolic complications after enterocystoplasty was very low [149]. None of the reported cases had acute problems during pregnancy.

Neobladder

As the authors have shown in an analysis, female sexuality does not have to be impaired by cystectomy and formation of an ileal neobladder. Especially in patients with interstitial cystitis, the lack of pain during intercourse may improve significantly the patient's sexual life [2]. To date, there is only one reported case of pregnancy in a patient with a neobladder, and she was treated at the authors' institution [150]. She had a partial agenesis of the os sacrum and neurogenic bladder. At age 2, she had an ileal conduit, followed by recurrent problems with stomal stenosis and hydronephrosis, requiring several operations. At age 20, it was decided to perform undiversion to an ileal neobladder. The patient has performed clean intermittent catheterization five to six times per day since then. Five years later, the patient became pregnant and had an uneventful course of pregnancy. She underwent cesarean section at 38 weeks of gestation. The intraoperative finding revealed a mesentery of the neobladder pushed to the right side by the growing uterus. The continence mechanism was not damaged by pregnancy or delivery.

Delivery

In all patients with urinary diversion, the form of delivery must be planned considering many relevant aspects, including potential damage to the urinary diversion by cesarean section, potential damage to the pelvic floor by vaginal delivery, special anatomic problems of the mother, and problems of the child.

Vaginal delivery

The pelvic floor has three important functions: supportive, sphincteric, and sexual functioning [151]. Vaginal delivery causes partial denervation of the pelvic floor in 80% of women delivering their first child [152]. Childbirth may result in pelvic support defects, problems with urinary continence, and sexual dysfunction. The damage results from direct damage and stretching effects to the muscle fibers of the vagina and pelvic floor and injury to the surrounding nerves [29]. Hill and Kramer [134] reported on 10 women with augmentation cystoplasties and native continence mechanisms who had vaginal delivery; 1 woman became incontinent after delivery. A case report described a patient who underwent subtotal cystectomy and ileal substitute bladder for interstitial cystitis, who later had vaginal delivery with vacuum extraction and developed urinary and fecal incontinence as a manifestation of a serious destabilization of the pelvic diaphragm [140]. In patients with ureterosigmoidostomy, any damage to the pelvic floor and the rectal continence mechanism may lead to a severe combined urinary and fecal incontinence. Vaginal delivery has the advantage, however, of avoiding any risk of injury to the mesenteric pedicle of the neobladder.

Vaginal delivery is contraindicated in the following patients:

Patients with a narrow bony pelvis
Patients with artificial sphincters or bladder neck reconstruction
Patients with contracted hips

Vaginal delivery should be performed with caution in the following patients:

Patients with ureterosigmoidostomy
Patients with malpresentation
Patients with cervical prolapse

Cesarean section

Hensle and associates [15] considered the elective scheduling of a cesarean delivery before the onset of labor the preferred method in patients with urinary diversion, in particular in patients with orthotopic continent urinary diversion. Hill and Kramer [134] had the same recommendation,

so that an experienced reconstructive urologist can be involved and have time to review thoroughly the patient's reconstructed anatomy before the case.

It has been estimated that obstetric bladder injury occurs in 0.1 per 1000 vaginal deliveries and 1.4 per 1000 cesarean sections [153]. The obstetrician has to decide which of the different techniques for cesarean section to use in a given patient. Especially in orthotopic urinary diversions, it may be favorable to perform a high cesarean section to avoid any damage to the reservoir. Hensle and associates [15] recommended a cesarean section with a midline incision. In their series, the urinary reservoir or augmented bladder was pushed to the region from which the bowel segment was obtained to preserve the blood supply. In all cases, they found the reservoir to be easily moved away from the pregnant uterus. Hill and Kramer [134] reported on five women who had cesarean section after augmentation cystoplasty. One case was difficult because of multiple adhesions, but no mesenteric injuries occurred.

There are no contraindications against cesarean section, but it should be performed very cautiously in the following patients:

Patients with intraperitoneal hydrocephalus shunts
Patients with pouches, enterocystoplasties, or neobladders

Special aspects

*Which form of urinary diversion
should be recommended in young patients
who plan to have children?*

As this review of the literature shows, a successful course of pregnancy is possible with all types of urinary diversion. The authors strongly recommend that the choice of the type of urinary diversion should consider first the individual situation and needs of the patient, but with secondary consideration for a potential pregnancy.

Is simultaneous sterilization an option?

In the early twentieth century, most patients with urinary diversion had simultaneous sterilization. The first patients who became pregnant after urinary diversion did so despite sterilization. Today, sterilization of patients undergoing urinary diversion is not performed routinely because pregnancy is not considered contraindicated in patients with urinary diversion.

Are there medical indications for an interruption?

In 1972, Olesen [108] recommended a therapeutic abortion, if the renal function was abnormal, when pregnancy was diagnosed. Because the possibilities of saving the renal function during pregnancy have greatly improved with modern medical care, this general recommendation should be obsolete in 2006.

What examinations are recommended before, during, and after pregnancy?

Richmond and coworkers [39] suggested that, whenever possible, counseling of patients with myelomeningocele should be done before conception, when radiologic pelvimetry and renal function assessment could be performed without risk to the fetus in utero. All pregnant women with any type of urinary diversion should be assessed (ideally antepartum) by a multidisciplinary team of experts, involving the obstetrician (perinatologist), urologist, obstetric anesthesiologist, general surgeon, neonatologist, and nursing staff who work together to tailor the optimal peripartum plan on a case-by-case basis [53]. Kennedy and colleagues [21] recommended an initial screening maternal ultrasound examination at 20 weeks of gestation to look for maternal hydronephrosis. Follow-up maternal renal ultrasound should be performed if hydronephrosis is noted initially or for recurrent episodes of pyleonephritis. In Germany, the patient is seen by the obstetrician every 4 weeks during the first 4 months of gestation, every 3 weeks during the next 3 months, every 2 weeks during the next 2 months, and then in weekly intervals until delivery. The authors strongly recommend that the patient see a urologist at the same intervals. The urologist should perform urinalysis, urine culture, and renal ultrasound (including estimation of the resistive index when hydronephrosis is present) and evaluate the storage function and emptying of the urinary diversion.

What information on reconstructive urology does an obstetrician need?

The obstetrician needs complete information on the anatomic situation of a patient with urinary diversion. Knowledge of all reports on previous surgical procedures performed in this particular patient is compulsory. Precise information on the fixation points of the urinary diversion and on the course of the ureters is necessary. Urologic input at the time of surgery aids identification of the lower urinary tract anatomy, prompt recognition of any advertent urinary tract injury, and assistance in the repair of any damage.

Is long-term antibiotic prophylaxis needed during pregnancy with a urinary diversion?

Symptomatic urinary tract infection is a problem in a large proportion of patients with urinary diversion. Contributing factors to urinary tract infections are urinary stasis, difficulty with clean intermittent catheterization, and ureteric compression. In one series, 21% of the patients reviewed had premature labor, presumably related to the high incidence of lower urinary tract infections and acute episodes of pyelonephritis. The authors advocated aggressive antibiotic therapy for all urinary tract infections in this group of patients [54]. Hensle and colleagues [15] also recommended maintaing all these women on antibiotic prophylaxis throughout pregnancy. The authors believe that low-dose antibiotic prophylaxis is at least advisable in the following patients:

Patients with a history of feverish urinary tract infection during pregnancy
Patients with hydronephrosis
Patients with impaired renal function
Patients with ureteral reflux
Patients with catheterization
Patients with ureterosigmoidostomy

Can successful pregnancy occur after urinary diversion and renal transplantation?

The first successful pregnancy after renal transplantation ended in 1958 with the delivery of a healthy child [154]. Since then, a growing number of reports on successful pregnancies have been published. Problems such as immunosuppression, impaired renal function, and obstructive uropathy may lead to a much less favorable prognosis for pregnancy in transplant patients compared with patients with urinary diversion alone. To date, only three pregnancies in women with a kidney transplanted to an ileal conduit were reported. In two cases, pregnancy had to be terminated at 10 and 22 weeks of gestation because of progressing renal failure from compression of the ileal loop [110]. The only successful pregnancy was published by Hein and colleagues [104]. Their patient had a neurogenic bladder from occult spina bifida. At age 14, an ileal conduit was created. Nine years later, she had progressive renal failure from chronic pyelonephritis and underwent bilateral nephrectomy. At the age of 26, a living donor kidney transplantation was performed. Four months later, the patient became pregnant. At 35 weeks of gestation, an intermittent obstruction of the left ureter was noted, leading to the decision of terminating the pregnancy. Delivery of a healthy boy was accomplished by a low segment cesarean section because of a narrow pelvic cavity. The postoperative course was uneventful.

Are pregnancy tests accurate in patients with urinary diversion?

Nethercliffe and coworkers [155] analyzed urine of patients with urinary diversion using the Clearview pregnancy test (Unipath Ltd. Bedford, England). Although all of these patients were not pregnant, positive pregnancy tests were found in 8 women and 5 men (false-positive rate 57%). These authors suggested that the mucus produced in enterocystoplasties may interfere with the pregnancy test. Patients have to be aware of this.

References

[1] Stein R, Hohenfellner K, Fisch M, et al. Social integration, sexual behaviour and fertility in patients with bladder exstrophy—a long-term follow up. Eur J Pediatr 1996;155:678–83.

[2] Volkmer BG, Gschwend JE, Herkommer K, et al. Cystectomy and orthotopic ileal neobladder: the impact on female sexuality. J Urol 2004;172:2353–7.

[3] Burbige KA, Hensle TW, Chambers WJ, et al. Pregnancy and sexual function in women with bladder exstrophy. Urology 1986;28:12–4.

[4] Solman F. Pregnancy in the woman with a stoma. Midwife Health Visit Community Nurse 1987;23:150–2.

[5] Van Horn C, Barrett P. Pregnancy, delivery, and postpartum experiences of fifty-four women with ostomies. J Wound Ostomy Continence Nurs 1997;24:151–62.

[6] Knauf AR. The late results of operations for the cure of exstrophy of the bladder. Papers from the Mayo Foundation and Medical School, University of Minnesota 1922;2:168–70.

[7] Kohler FP. Management of pregnancy following lower urinary tract diversion. Am J Obstet Gynecol 1967;97:1149–50.

[8] Krisiloff M, Puchner PJ, Treter W, et al. Pregnancy in women with bladder exstrophy. J Urol 1978;119:478–9.

[9] Loughlin KR. Management of urologic problems during pregnancy. Urology 1994;44:159–69.

[10] Barron WM. The pregnant surgical patient: medical evaluation and management. Ann Intern Med 1984;101:683–91.

[11] Gogarten W, Marcus MA, Van Aken H. Gynäkologie und Geburtshilfe. In: Kochs E, Krier C, Buzello W, Adams HA, editors. Anästhesiologie. New York: Thieme; 2001. p. 1008–23.

[12] Pitkin RM. Morphologic changes in pregnancy. In: Buchsbaum HJ, Schmidt JD, editors. Gynecologic and obstetric urology. Philadelphia: Saunders; 1993. p. 581–8.

[13] Robertson EG. Alterations in renal function during pregnancy. In: Buchsbaum HJ, Schmidt JD, editors. Gynecologic and obstetric urology. Philadelphia: Saunders; 1993. p. 607–20.

[14] Akerlund S, Bokström H, Jonsson O, et al. Pregnancy and delivery in patients with urinary diversion through the continent ileal reservoir. Surg Gynecol Obstet 1991;173:350–2.

[15] Hensle TW, Bingham JB, Reiley EA, et al. The urologic care and outcome of pregnancy after urinary tract reconstruction. BJU Int 2004;93:588–90.

[16] Kretschew KP. Intestinal stoma. Philadelphia: Saunders; 1972. p. 281–3.

[17] Hudson CN. Ileostomy in pregnancy. Proc R Soc Med 1972;65:281–3.

[18] Lennenberg ES. Modern concepts in the management of patients with intestinal and urinary stomas. Clin Obstet Gynaecol 1972;15:542–79.

[19] McEwan HP. Pregnancy in patients with surgically treated ulcerative colitis. J Obstet Gynaecol Br Commonw 1965;72:450–1.

[20] Loughlin KR, Kerr LA. The current management of urolithiasis during pregnancy. Urol Clin N Am 2002;29:701–4.

[21] Kennedy WA, Hensle TW, Reiley EA, et al. Pregnancy after orthotopic continent urinary diversion. Surg Gynecol Obstet 1993;177:405–9.

[22] Pedlow PRB. Pregnancy associated with ureterosigmoid anastomosis. J Obstet Gynaecol Br Commonw 1961;68:822–6.

[23] Valentin H. Schwangerschaft bei Vaginalstein und Exstrophie der Blase. Zbl Gynäkol 1958;80:1721–3.

[24] Overstreet EW, Hinman F Jr. Some gynecological aspects of bladder exstrophy with report of an illustrative case. West J Surg Obstet Gynecol 1956;64:131–7.

[25] Clemetson CAB. Ectopia vesicae and split pelvis. Br J Obstet Gynaecol 1958;65:973–81.

[26] Messelink EJ, Aronson DC, Knuist M, et al. Four cases of bladder exstrophy in two families. J Med Genet 1994;31:490–2.

[27] Ikeme ACC. Pregnancy in women after repair of bladder exstrophy. Br J Obstet Gynaecol 1981;88: 327–8.

[28] Grady RW, Mitchell ME. Bladder anomalies, exstrophy, and epispadias. In: Belman AB, King LR, Kramer SA, editors. Clinical pediatric urology. London: Martin Dunitz Ltd; 2002. p. 859–98.

[29] Pauls RN, Berman JR. Impact of pelvic floor disorders and prolapse on female sexual function and response. Urol Clin N Am 2002;29:677–83.

[30] Öjerskog B, Kock NG, Philipson BM, et al. Pregnancy and delivery in patients with a continent ileostomy. Surg Gynecol Obstet 1988;167:61–4.

[31] Stanton SL. Gynecologic complications of epispadias and bladder exstrophy. Am J Obstet Gynecol 1974;119:749–54.

[32] McGoogan LS. Pregnancy and urinary diversion. Pac Med Surg 1968;76:7–15.

[33] Daw E. Pregnancy problems in a paraplegic patient with an ileal conduit bladder. Practitioner 1973; 211:781–4.

[34] Robertson DNS. Pregnancy and labour in the paraplegic. Paraplegia 1972;10:209–12.

[35] Ellison FE. Term pregnancy in a patient with myelomeningocele, ureteroileostomy, and partial parapareses. Am J Obstet Gynecol 1975;123:33–4.

[36] Takagi H, Matsunami K, Imai A. Satisfactory pregnancy outcome in a patient with meningomyelocele. J Obstet Gynecol 2004;24:824–5.

[37] Rietberg CCT, Lindhout D. Adult patients with spina bifida cystica: genetic counselling, pregnancy and delivery. Eur J Obstet Gynaecol Reprod Biol 1993;52:63–70.

[38] Fujimoto A, Ebbin A, Wilson MG, et al. Successful pregnancy in a woman with meningomyelocele. Lancet 1973;13:104.

[39] Richmond D, Zabarievski I, Bond A. Management of pregnancy in mothers with spina bifida. Eur J Obstet Reprod Biol 1987;25:341–5.

[40] Wynn JS, Mellor S, Morewood GA. Pregnancy in patients with spina bifida cystica. Practitioner 1979;22:543–6.

[41] Robson WLM, Leung AKC, Sinclair OJ. Congenital urinary abnormalities and neural tube defect. Child Nephrol Urol 1991;11:84–6.

[42] Meeropol E, Kelleher R, Bell S, et al. Allergic reactions to rubber in patients with myelodysplasia. N Engl J Med 1990;323:1072.

[43] Slater JE, Mostello LA, Shear C. Rubber specific IgE in children with spina bifida. J Urol 1991;146: 578–9.

[44] Stein SC, Schut L. Hydrocephalus in myelomeningocele. Childs Brain 1979;5:413–9.

[45] Greenberg MS. Handbook of neurosurgery. 5th edition. New York: Thieme; 2001. p. 153–4.

[46] Wisoff JH, Kratzert KJ, Handwerker SM. Pregnancy in patients with cerebrospinal fluid shunts: report of a series and review of the literature. Neurosurgery 1991;29:827–31.

[47] Hanakita J, Suzuki T, Yamamoto Y, et al. Ventriculoperitoneal shunt malfunction during pregnancy. J Neurosurg 1985;63:459–60.

[48] Cusimano MD, Meffe FM, Gentili F, et al. Ventriculoperitoneal shunt malfunction during pregnancy. Neurosurgery 1990;27:969–71.

[49] Monfared AH, Koh KS, Apuzzo MLJ, et al. Obstetric management of pregnant women with extracranial shunts. J Can Med Assoc 1979; 120:562–3.

[50] Gast MJ, Grubb RL, Stickler RC. Maternal hydrocephalus and pregnancy. Obstet Gynecol 1983;62: 29S–31S.

[51] Kleinman G, Sutherling W, Martinez M, et al. Malfunction of ventriculoperitoneal shunts during pregnancy. Obstet Gynecol 1983;61:753–4.

[52] Asif A, Uehling DT. Successful pregnancy following ureteroileostomy. Am J Obstet Gynecol 1969; 105:641–2.

[53] Kuczkowski KM, Hay B. Peripartum care of the parturient with Indiana continent urinary diversion: a need for a multidisciplinary approach. Ann Fr Anesth Reanim 2004;23:927–8.

[54] Barrett RJ, Peters WA. Pregnancy following urinary diversion. Obstet Gynecol 1983;62:582–6.

[55] Lattimer JK, Beck L, Yeaw S. Long-term followup after exstrophy closure: late improvement and good quality of life. J Urol 1978;119:864–6.

[56] Hoch WH, Shanser JD, Burns RA. Ureterosigmoidostomy: a 59-year followup and review of long-term urinary diversion. J Urol 1979;122: 407–8.

[57] Vordermark JS, Deshon GE, Agee RE. Management of pregnancy after major urinary tract reconstruction. Obstet Gynecol 1990;75:564–7.

[58] Akaza H, Komine Y, Ueno A, et al. Long-term survival with experience of normal delivery after ureterosigmoidostomy: a case report. Nippon Hinyokika Gakkai Zasshi 1978;69:1104–8.

[59] Antakova LA. Povtornaia dososhennaia beremennost' posle operatsii peresadki mochetochnikov v priamuiu kishku po povodu ekstrofii mochevogo puzyria. Urol Nefrol (Mosk) 1966;31:44–5.

[60] Battke H, Woraschk HJ. Schwangerschaft und Geburt nach Coffey-Mayo-Operation. Zentralbl Gynakol 1963;85:1576–9.

[61] Cabot H. Treatment of exstrophy of the bladder. N Engl J Med 1931;205:707.

[62] De Luca P, Torella M, Festa B. Gravidanza complicata da ISO-Rh in paziente nata con estrofia vesicale ed operata di impianto sigmoideo degli ureteri. Arch Ostet Ginecol 1982;87:203–13.

[63] Eberbach CW, Pierce JM. Pregnancy terminated by caesarean section after ureteral transplantation into the sigmoid. Surg Gynecol Obstet 1928;47: 540–2.

[64] Farkas G, Bältescu W. Schwangerschafts- und Geburtsverlauf nach Harnleiter-Darm-Anastomose. Zentralbl Chir 1968;93:1609–14.

[65] Green-Armytage VB. Complete exstrophy of the bladder with split pelvis. J Obstet Gynaecol Br Emp 1926;33:469.

[66] Hinman F Jr. Concerning pregnancy after ureter-ointestinal anastomosis. Am J Obstet Gynecol 1951;62:192.

[67] Hoehne G. Spontangeburt nach Coffey-Mayo-Operation. Geburtsh u Frauenheilkd 1957;17:1063.

[68] Hung C, Jesurun HM. Pregnancy in a patient with ureterosigmoid anastomosis. J Med Soc N J 1970; 67:259–60.

[69] Kiliam A, Grillo D, Summerson DJ. Pregnancy and delivery after uretero-sigmoidostomy. Am J Obstet Gynecol 1967;97:278.

[70] Kohler FP. Pregnancy in the presence of lower urinary tract diversion. J Urol 1967;97:683.

[71] Lanman TH. Treatment of exstrophy of the bladder. Postgrad Med 1950;7:129.

[72] Ledfors GE, Lansing JD, Slate WG, et al. Pregnancy and exstrophy of the urinary bladder. Obstet Gynecol 1966;28:254–7.

[73] Lotimer LE. Pregnancy and delivery following bilateral ureterosigmoid transplant for exstrophy of the bladder. Am J Obstet Gynecol 1954;67:28.

[74] Lower WE. Disposition of ureters in certain abnormal conditions of the urinary bladder. JAMA 1923; 29:1200.

[75] Movers F. Geburt bei angeborenem Spaltbecken und operierter Blasenektopie. Geburtsh u Frauenheil 1951;11:247–51.

[76] Nabity SF. Pregnancy and delivery following bilateral ureteral transplant to the bowel for exstrophy of the bladder: report of a case. Nebr State Med J 1966;51:284–6.

[77] Nicolich G. Considerazioni sui resultati lontani della ureterosigmoidostomia. Minerva Med 1977; 68:1925–7.

[78] Pietsch P, Lober R, Würfel S. Gynäkologisch-geburtshilfliche Probleme bei Patientinnen mit Harnleiter-Darm-Anastomose nach Blasenekstrophie. Zbl Gynäkol 1983;105:1450–6.

[79] Plym-Florshell Y. Ein Fall von Ektopia vesicae operata mit mehreren späteren Komplikationen. Acta Path Microbiol Scand Suppl 1953;16:350–7.

[80] Randall LM, Hardwick RD. Pregnancy and parturition following bilateral ureteral transplantation for congenital exstrophy of the bladder. Surg Gynecol Obstet 1934;58:1018–20.

[81] Richter K. Schwangerschaft und Geburt nach Coffey-Mayo'scher Operation wegen Spaltblase. Wien Med Wochen 1962;112:541–5.

[82] Roloff. Zbl Chir 1924;44:2432.

[83] Schnecke G. Schwangerschaft und Spontangeburt nach Coffey-Operation wegen Ekstrophia vesicae. Zbl Gynäkol 1966;88:220–2.

[84] Scholz A. Schwangerschaft und Geburt nach Nephrektomie und Coffey-Mayo-Operation wegen Nierentuberkulose. Zbl Gynäkol 1958;80:496–501.

[85] Schraeder H. Dissertation, Universität Düsseldorf; 1958.

[86] Schumann H. Schwangerschaft bei einer wegen angeborener Blasenektopie mit Spaltbecken operierten 25jährigen Frau. Geburtsh u Frauenheil 1942;4:318–33.

[87] Smythe AR. Pregnancy associated with exstrophy of the bladder, obstructive renal failure, and vaginal hysterotomy. Annual Meeting Armed Forces District of the American College of Obstetricians and Gynecologists. Orlando (FL), October 5–10, 1980.

[88] Suhler A, Duplay H, Commandre F, et al. Grossesse à évolution favorable 24 ans après urétéro-sigmoidostomie pour estrophie vésicale, malgré un traitement prolongé par chloraminophéne et corticoides pour polyarthrite chronique évolutive. J Urol Nephrol (Paris) 1973;79:599–604.

[89] Turner GG. The treatment of congenital defects of the bladder and urethra by implantation of the ureters into the bowel: with a record of 17 personal cases. Br J Surg 1929;17:114–78.

[90] Voges GE, Orestano L, Schumacher S, et al. Kontinente Harnableitung und Schwangerschaft. Geburtsh u Frauenheilk 1995;55:711–5.

[91] Volkmer BG, Seidl EM, Gschwend JE, et al. Pregnancy in women with ureterosigmoidostomy. Urology 2002;60:979–82.

[92] Wesolowsky S, Bulska M. Pregnancy after ureterosigmoid anastomosis. Gynaecologia 1956; 141:56.

[93] Zeffer J, Gyarmathy F. Egyveséjü asszony terhessége és szülése ureterosigmoidostomia után 13 évvel. Orv Hetil 1968;109:535–6.

[94] Koelliker SL, Cronan JJ. Acute urinary tract obstruction—imaging update. Urol Clin N Am 1997;24:571–82.

[95] Goodwin WE, Scardino PT. Ureterosigmoidostomy. J Urol 1977;118:169–74.

[96] Benson JT. Pregnancy after ureterosigmoid anastomosis. Obstet Gynecol 1966;27:294.

[97] Bravo RH, Katz M. Ureteral obstruction in a pregnant patient with an ileal loop conduit: a case report. J Reprod Med 1983;28:427–9.

[98] Cass AS, Bloom BA, Luxenberg M. Sexual function in adults with myelomeningocele. J Urol 1986;136:425–6.

[99] Ehrenberg HM, Mercer BM, Catalano P, et al. Pregnancy in a spinal cord-injured bilateral total leg amputee: management and considerations. Am J Obstet Gynecol 2003;188:1096–9.

[100] Nash E, quoted by Hudson CN. Ileostomy in pregnancy. Proc R Soc Med 1972;65:281–3.

[101] Feitz WFJ, Van Grunsven EJKJEM, Froeling FMJA, et al. Outcome analysis of the psychosexual and socioeconomical development of adult patients born with bladder exstrophy. J Urol 1994;152: 1417–9.

[102] Gontero P, Masood S, Sogni F, et al. Upper urinary tract complications in pregnant women with an ileal conduit. Scand J Urol Nephrol 2004;38:523–4.

[103] Greenberg RE, Vaughn ED, Pitts WR. Normal pregnancy and delivery after ileal conduit urinary diversion. J Urol 1981;125:172–3.

[104] Hein PR, Jansen JLJ, Debruyne FMJ. Successful pregnancy after renal transplantation in a patient with a urinary diversion. Eur J Obstet Gynaecol Reprod Biol 1978;8:129–32.

[105] Mann WJ, Jones DED. Pregnancy complicated by maternal neural tube defect and an ileal conduit: a case report. J Reprod Med 1976;17:339–41.

[106] Miller GD, Slade PJB. Successful pregnancy in a patient with previous ectopia vesicae. Br J Urol 1978;50:281.

[107] Natarajan V, Kapur D, Sharma S, et al. Pregnancy in patients with spina bifida and urinary diversion. Int Urogynecol J 2002;13:383–5.

[108] Olesen S. Pregnancy complicated by ureteroileocutaneostomy. Dan Med Bull 1972;19:108–9.

[109] Powell B, Garvey M. Complications of maternal spina bifida. Ir J Med Sci 1984;153:20–1.

[110] Sciarra JJ, Toledo-Pereyra LH, Bendel RP, et al. Pregnancy following renal transplantation. Am J Obstet Gynecol 1975;123:411–25.

[111] Singh G, Wilkinson JM, Thomas DG. Supravesical diversion for incontinence: a long-term follow up. Br J Urol 1997;70:348–53.

[112] Makkas. Zbl Chir 1910;33:1073.

[113] Forshell YP. Ein Fall von Ektopia vesicae operata mit mehreren späteren Komplikationen. 350–7.

[114] Hatch TR, Steinberg RW, Davis LE. Successful term delivery by cesarean section in a patient with a continent ileocecal urinary diversion. J Urol 1991;146:1111–2.

[115] Schumacher S, Fichtner J, Stein R, et al. Pregnancy after Mainz pouch urinary diversion. J Urol 1997; 158:1362–4.

[116] Sharma D, Singhal SR, Singhal SK. Successful pregnancy in a patient with previous bladder exstrophy. Aust N Z J Obstet Gynaecol 1998;38:227–8.

[117] Thaly R, Chernoff A. Pregnancy in a patient with an Indiana pouch. J Urol 2004;172:200.

[118] Wiedemann A, Thüroff J, Venn HJ. Harnblasenersatz und Schwangerschaft. Akt Urol 1993;5:291–2.

[119] Greenwell TJ, Venn SN, Creighton S, et al. Pregnancy after lower urinary tract reconstruction for congenital abnormalities. BJU Int 2003;92:773–7.

[120] Von Mikulicz J. Zur Operation der angeborenen Blasenspalte. Zbl Chir 1889;20:641–3.

[121] Couvelaire R. La petite vessie des tuberculeux genitourinaires: essai de classification, places et variantes des cysto-intestinoplasties. J Urol (Paris) 1950;56:381–434.

[122] Smith RB, van Cangh P, Skinner DG, et al. Augmentation enterocystoplasty: a critical review. J Urol 1977;118:35–9.

[123] Adams MC, Mitchell MD, Rink RC. Gastrocystoplasty: an alternative solution to the problem of urological reconstruction in the severely compromised patient. J Urol 1988;140:1152–6.

[124] Bruce PT, Wheelahan JB, Buckham GJ. "Undiversion" with colocystoplasty for neurogenic bladder: a report of 2 cases. Br J Urol 1979;51:269–74.

[125] Chosson J, Ruf H, Ayme Y. Tuberculose rénale et grossesse. Bull Fed Gynecol Obstet Franc 1962;14: 157–9.

[126] Cibert J, Pigeaud H, Cibert J. Iléo-cystoplastie et grossesse. J Urol Med Chir 1959;65:421–3.

[127] Corthout EP. Néovessie et grossesse: revue de la littérature et présentation de 2 cas. Bull Soc R Belge Gynecol Obstet 1968;38:479–84.

[128] Cvetkovic B. Trudnoca i porodaj kod vezikoileoplastike. Acta Chir Jugosl 1961;8:198–202.

[129] Doyle BA, Smith SP, Stempel LE. Urinary undiversion and pregnancy. Am J Obstet Gynecol 1988; 158:1131–2.

[130] Foret J, Gregoire L. Sur un cas d'uretero-cysto-iléoplastie suivie d'une grossesse menée à terme. Bull Soc R Belge Gynecol Obstet 1955;26: 168–71.

[131] Garcia Rodriguez-Acosta V. Embarazo a termino y parto espontaneo en una operada de colocistoplastia. Arch Esp Urol 1963;16:211–3.

[132] Goodwin WE, Betenbaugh HS, Haynes VE, et al. Full-term pregnancy and spontaneous delivery after ileocystoplasty. JAMA 1962;181:906–8.

[133] Hill DE, Chantigian PM, Kramer SA. Pregnancy after augmentation cystoplasty. Surg Gynecol Obstet 1990;170:485.

[134] Hill DE, Kramer SA. Management of pregnancy after augmentation cystoplasty. J Urol 1990;144: 457–9.

[135] Lebrun J. Iléo-cystoplastie et grossesse. J Urol Nephrol (Paris) 1965;71:94–7.

[136] Mori Y, Wakitani TA. A spontaneous delivery at 36 weeks' gestation after ileocystoplasty. Mie Med J 1967;17:133–9.

[137] Okolicany O, Hatvany T, Sochor J, et al. L'observation d'une grossesse après une iléo-cystoplastie. J Urol Nephrol (Paris) 1964;70:91–4.

[138] Perrin J, Lyonnet R, Verrier JP, et al. Iléocystoplastie pour tuberculose rénale, grossesse gémelläire, accouchement par les voies naturelles sans difficulté spéciale. Bull Fed Soc Gynecol Obstet 1966;18: 38–9.

[139] Pigeaud H, Cibert J, Neumann E. Deuxième observation de grossesse après iléo-cystoplastie. Bull Fed Gynecol Obstet Franc 1961;13:306.

[140] Schilling A, Krawczak G, Friesen A, et al. Pregnancy in a patient with an ileal substitute bladder followed by severe destabilization of the pelvic support. J Urol 1996;155:1389–90.

[141] Taniguchi A, Kakizaki H, Murakumo M, et al. Management of pregnancy and delivery after

augmentation cystoplasty. Nippon Hinyokika Gakkai Zasshi 2002;93:39–43.

[142] Truc E, Durand G, Henriet R. Issue favorable d'une grossesse après iléo-cystoplastie. J Urol Med Chir 1960;66:791–2.

[143] Uhlir K. Contribution à l'evolution de la grossesse aprés entéro-cysto- ou urétéroplastie. J Urol Nephrol (Paris) 1967;73:681–6.

[144] Turner-Warwick R, Ashken MH. The functional results of partial, subtotal and total cystoplasty with special reference to enterocystoplasty, selective sphincterotomy and cystocystoplasty. Br J Urol 1967;39:3–12.

[145] Smith AM. Enterocystoplasty and pregnancy. Am J Obstet Gynecol 1973;117:527.

[146] Khoury JM, Timmons SL, Corbel L. Complications of enterocystoplasty. J Urol 1992;40:9–14.

[147] Creagh TA, McInerney PD, Thomas PJ. Pregnancy after lower urinary tract reconstruction in women. J Urol 1995;154:1323–4.

[148] Gilbert SM, Hensle TW. Metabolic consequences and long-term complications of enterocystoplasty in children: a review. J Urol 2005;173:1080–3.

[149] Blaivas JG, Weiss JP, Desai P, et al. Long-term followup of augmentation enterocystoplasty and continent diversion in patients with benign disease. J Urol 2005;173:1631–4.

[150] Volkmer BG. Neue Aspekte der Zystektomie im Neoblasen-Zeitalter. Habilitationsschrift, Universität Ulm; 2005.

[151] Wallace K. Female pelvic floor functions, dysfunctions and behavioral approaches to treatment. Clin Sports Med 1994;13:459–81.

[152] Allen RE, Hosker GL, Smith AR, et al. Pelvic floor damage and childbirth: a neurophysiologic study. Br J Obstet Gynaecol 1990;97: 770–9.

[153] Rajasekar D, Hall M. Urinary tract injuries during obstetric intervention. Br J Obstet Gynaecol 1997; 104:731–4.

[154] Murray JE, Reid DE, Harrison JH, et al. Successful pregnancies after human renal transplantation. N Engl J Med 1963;269:341.

[155] Nethercliffe J, Trewick A, Samuell C, et al. False-positive pregnancy tests in patients with enterocystoplasties. BJU Int 2001;87:780–2.

ELSEVIER
SAUNDERS

Urol Clin N Am 34 (2007) 89–101

UROLOGIC
CLINICS
of North America

Current Diagnosis and Management of Fetal Genitourinary Abnormalities

Katherine C. Hubert, MD[a], Jeffrey S. Palmer, MD, FACS, FAAP[b],*

[a]Case Western Reserve University 11100 Euclid Avenue Cleveland, OH 44106, USA
[b]Glickman Urological Institute, Children's Hospital at Cleveland Clinic and Cleveland Clinic Lerner College of
Medicine of Case Western Reserve University, 9500 Euclid Avenue, A100, Cleveland, OH 44195, USA

Ultrasonography is an essential tool for the prenatal diagnosis and monitoring of fetal genitourinary abnormalities. Helin and Per-Haken evaluated the frequency of urinary tract anomalies by routine prenatal ultrasonography in almost 12,000 pregnant patients [1]. They found an overall frequency of fetal malformations of 0.5%, approximately half of which were abnormalities of the urinary tract. As expected, the ability to detect major genitourinary anomalies has impacted the outcome of pregnancies. Cromie and colleagues reviewed pregnancy termination rates of fetuses with spina bifida, posterior urethral valves (PUV), prune belly syndrome, and exstrophy over a 20-year period [2]. They found that pregnancy was electively terminated because of spina bifida (65% of cases), PUV (46% of cases), prune belly syndrome (31% of cases), and exstrophy (25% of cases). In those cases where termination of the pregnancy is not selected, early detection of anomalies by ultrasonography allows for appropriately timed intervention in cases where there is potential to preserve renal function.

Prenatal assessment with ultrasonography provides excellent imaging of fluid-filled structures (eg, hydronephrosis, renal cysts, and dilated bladder) and renal parenchyma. This information allows for the generation of a differential diagnosis, identification of associated anomalies, and assessment of the prenatal and postnatal risks of a given anomaly. This enhances for parental education and prenatal and postnatal planning. This article discusses current methods of diagnosis and management of fetal genitourinary anomalies, and also the postnatal evaluation and treatment of these conditions.

Hydronephrosis: general considerations for evaluation and management

Routine prenatal ultrasonography, usually performed at 16 to 20 weeks, has revealed many cases of in utero hydronephrosis. Prenatal hydronephrosis, the most common prenatal genitourinary ultrasonographic abnormality, can result in a significant amount of parental stress. The ability for the health care provider to help reduce this stress is based on an understanding of the differential diagnoses and their ramifications. The differential diagnoses can range from a self-limited condition without clinical significance (ie, physiologic hydronephrosis with a normal ultrasonogram postnatally) to conditions that require surgical intervention (eg, ureteropelvic junction [UPJ] obstruction), to renal destruction and involution (eg, multicystic dysplastic kidney). Therefore, it is important for the urologist and obstetrician to understand the differential diagnoses with the associated findings and clinical implications to accurately relate this information to the parents.

Important factors to consider in the assessment of hydronephrosis include fetal wellbeing, gestational age, unilaterality versus bilaterality, and amniotic fluid volume. Box 1 lists the differential diagnoses of hydronephrosis, and Table 1 explains these diagnoses in more detail.

* Corresponding author.
  E-mail address: palmerjs@ccf.org
(J.S. Palmer).

**Box 1. Differential diagnoses
of hydronephrosis**

UPJ obstruction
Vesicoureteral reflux (VUR)
Primary nonrefluxing megaureter
Ureterocele
Ureterovesical junction (UVJ)
    obstruction
Ectopic ureter
Posterior urethral valves
Megacystis megaureter
Physiologic dilatation
Multicystic dysplastic kidney
Autosomal recessive polycystic kidney
    disease
Exstrophy
Prune belly syndrome

Diagnosis of hydronephrosis

The threshold for the diagnosis of hydronephrosis is based on the recognition that renal pelvic diameter may vary with gestational age. There is considerable variation in the definition of prenatal hydronephrosis in the literature. Siemens and colleagues found that an anteroposterior diameter (APD) of the fetal renal pelvis measuring greater than 6 mm at less than 20 weeks, greater than 8mm at 20 to 30 weeks, and greater than 10 mm at greater than 30 weeks was associated with persistent postnatal renal abnormalities [3]. Stocks and colleagues diagnosed hydronephrosis when fetal APD was 4 mm or greater before 33 weeks of gestation, or 7 mm or greater at or after 33 weeks of gestation [4]. Using these criteria, they found a statistically significant difference in APD at study entry between patients with a postnatal diagnosis of UPJ obstruction (11.19 +/− 1.24 mm) and those with normal kidneys postnatally (7.07 +/− 0.58 mm). There was no significant difference for this measurement when normal patients were compared with those with a postnatal diagnosis of VUR (7.94 +/− 1.21 mm) or extrarenal pelvis (9.19 +/− 1.35 mm). No correlation was noted between increasing APD (defined as 2 mm or more) on successive prenatal ultrasonography and postnatal outcome. Decreasing prenatal APD did not predict the absence of hydronephrosis or a normal outcome postnatally. Based on stricter criteria for prenatal hydronephrosis, Docimo and colleagues found that in 101 neonates who had hydronephrosis on

prenatal ultrasonography (defined as APD ≥4 mm at <20 weeks, APD ≥5 mm at 20 to 26 weeks, APD ≥6 mm at 27 to 35 weeks and APD ≥7 mm at 36 or more weeks), 59 (58%) had a normal neonatal ultrasonography or mild hydronephrosis [5]. Low-grade prenatal mydronephrosis has a much greater chance of resolution than high-grade hydronephrosis [6].

After 20 weeks of gestation, prenatal hydronephrosis is assessed using the commonly used grading system [7]:

- Grade 1—pelvic APD of 1 cm and no caliectasis
- Grade 2—pelvic APD of 1 to 1.5 cm and no caliectasis
- Grade 3—pelvic APD is greater than 1.5 cm and slight caliectasis
- Grade 4—pelvic APD is greater than 1.5 cm and moderate caliectasis
- Grade 5—pelvic APD is greater than 1.5 cm and severe caliectasis and cortical atrophy (cortex <2 mm thick)

The total volume of amniotic fluid, which ranges from 500 to 2000 mL, is also an important factor in a fetus with hydronephrosis. In early gestation, the source of amniotic fluid is a transudate of maternal plasma [8]. By 16 weeks, most amniotic fluid is fetal urine. The volume increases until the end of the second trimester at a relative constant rate, then it remains steady, and then decreases shortly before term [9]. Oligohydramnios refers to a reduced amount of amniotic fluid, which been shown to result in pulmonary maldevelopment and somatic compression [10].

Prenatal hydronephrosis may be caused by various obstructive and nonobstructive etiologies. Kaefer and colleagues evaluated increased renal echogenicity as a sonographic sign for differentiation between obstructive and nonobstructive etiologies of fetal bladder distention [11]. They evaluated 18 male fetuses with bilateral hydronephrosis and bladder distention that were diagnosed with PUV, megacystitis–megaureter association, or prune belly syndrome postnatally. They found that the criteria of oligohydramnios and increased renal echogenicity were highly predictive of an obstructive etiology with a sensitivity of 100% and a specificity of 93%. This has implications for prenatal and postnatal management, as the fetus with an obstructive etiology may be a candidate for prenatal intervention (eg, vesicoamniotic shunt.).

Other studies have evaluated the prognostic value of various criteria used to assess functional

Table 1
Elements of prenatal urologic ultrasonographic diagnosis

Parameter	Comment	Possible causes
Hydronephrosis	Variable severity; may include pelviectasis and/or caliectasis	Obstruction, reflux
Caliectasis	Intrarenal dilation; more indicative of significant pathologic process	Obstruction, reflux
Pelvic anterior–posterior diameter	Measured in the coronal plane, variable; in extremes may predict clinical outcome; caution should be exercised in over-reliance on these measurements	Increased in obstruction, reflux
Renal parenchyma	Echogenicity should be less than liver or spleen; lucent medullary pyramids should be seen	Increased echogenicity in dysplasia, obstruction, ARPKD
Urothelial thickening	Increased thickness of pelvic lining	Variable dilation as with reflux or occasionally obstruction
Duplication	Separation of renal pelvic sinus echoes when no hydronephrosis seen	Possible associated reflux or obstruction; look for dilated ureter and ureterocele
Cystic structures, renal	Simple cysts rare	MCDK, ADPKD
Cystic structures, intravesical	May be very large and fill bladder; thin-walled	Ureterocele
Urinoma	Fluid collection around kidney; perinephric or subcapsular	Obstruction
Bladder filling	Fill and void cycles may be demonstrated over time	Urine production
Bladder wall thickness	Must be interpreted in context of bladder filling	Obstruction, neurogenic dysfunction
"keyhole sign"	Dilated posterior urethral; difficult to image	Posterior urethral valves
Oligohydramnios	Markedly reduced amniotic fluid; usually considered as no pocket of fluid <2 cm	Poor urine output due to obstruction and/or renal failure

Abbreviations: ARPKD, autosomal recessive polycystic kidney disease; MCDK, multicystic dysplastic kidney.
From Peters CA. Perinatal urology. In: Walsh PC, Retik AB, Vaughan ED, et al, eds. Campbell's Urology. 8th ed. Philadelphia: WB Saunders, 2002; with permission.

potential for normal renal and pulmonary function at birth in fetuses with bilateral congenital hydronephrosis. Glick and colleagues reviewed the management of 20 fetuses with congenital hydronephrosis. Of the 20, 19 had bladder outlet obstruction (caused by PUV or urethral atresia), and one had bilateral UPJ obstruction [12]. They classified the fetuses retrospectively into good outcome and poor outcome groups based on autopsy, biopsy, or clinical outcome. Their prognostic evaluation included amniotic fluid status at presentation, ultrasonographic evaluation of the renal parenchyma, and temporary bladder exteriorization to determine urine sodium and chloride concentrations, osmolarity, and urine output.

Fetal urine is made hypotonic by selective tubular reabsorption of sodium and chloride in excess of free water. Glick and colleagues found that the fetuses who later proved to have good function had normal hypotonic urine, whereas fetuses with poor function made isotonic urine. The group with good predicted function also had normal to moderately decreased amniotic fluid at the time of presentation, normal to echogenic sonographic appearance of the kidneys, and urine output of greater than 2 mL/h. They found no statistically significant difference between the two groups in fetal urine iothalamate excretion or potassium and creatinine concentrations. Cromblethorne and colleagues studied 40 fetuses referred for congenital bilateral hydronephrosis to assess the prognostic value of fetal urine electrolyte levels, osmolarity, and sonographic appearance of the kidneys [13]. They retrospectively assigned fetuses to a good prognosis group if fetal urine was hypotonic (sodium <100 mEq/L, chloride <90 mEq/L, and osmolarity <210 mOsm/L), and there was no evidence of renal dysplasia on ultrasonography. If one criterion was abnormal, fetuses were assigned to the poor prognosis group. They found that the prognostic criteria accurately predicted survival ($P < .005$) in fetuses who were candidates for intervention. Overall survival, excluding 14 elective terminations, was 16 of 26 (58%). In the poor prognosis group, overall survival, excluding elective terminations, was 3 of 10 (30%). Overall survival in the good prognosis group was 13 of 18 (81.2%). In six of the eight survivors in the good prognosis group, severe oligohydramnios was reversed by decompression. All of the survivors in the poor prognosis group required some form of fetal therapy. Based on the results of these studies, fetal urine electrolyte levels and ultrasonagraphic appearance of fetal kidneys may be helpful in predicting residual fetal renal function and neonatal outcome.

Fetal intervention

The overall benefit of therapeutic fetal intervention for hydronephrosis is controversial. Fetal intervention for hydronephrosis first was reported in the early 1980s. An open hysterotomy was performed to perform fetal urinary diversion. The infant was born at 35 weeks gestation, developed pulmonary hypoplasia, and did not survive [14]. Golbus and colleagues reported on the percutaneous placement of a vesicoamniotic shunt at 32 weeks gestation for prune belly syndrome [15]. At present, fetal intervention is indicated when oligohydramnios is present in association with bladder outlet obstruction (eg, PUV); there is a concern that the life of the neonate is at risk, and the fetus will benefit from in utero bladder decompression. Other factors that are required are a normal karyotype and a singleton pregnancy.

The technique for fetal vesicoamniotic shunt placement involves insertion of a double pigtail shunt under ultrasonographic guidance. These shunts thereby bypass the obstructed urethra [16]. Accurate placement of vesicoamniotic shunts can be difficult. More recently, endoscopic fetal intervention has been evolving as a newer treatment option to decompress the fetal bladder.

Quintero and colleagues described fetal cystoscopy and endoscopic valve ablation [17]. This technique requires further evaluation to determine if the fetal bladder is decompressed adequately.

Postnatal evaluation of hydronephrosis

Infants diagnosed with congenital hydronephrosis routinely undergo postnatal imaging evaluation. The optimal timing of postnatal ultrasonography and the criteria for voiding cystourethrography (VCUG) have been controversial. Because of the potential for false-negative results because of perinatal dehydration and lower glomerular filtration rate, postnatal ultrasonography to evaluate hydronephrosis typically is delayed for several days. Wiener and colleagues compared postnatal ultrasonography within 48 hours of birth to 7 to 10 days of life in 21 consecutive newborns with prenatal hydronephrosis, defined as a pelvic diameter at least 4 mm before 33 weeks gestation, or at least 8 mm after 33 weeks [18]. They found that 14 renal units had an increase in hydronephrosis between the first and second ultrasonograms, and eight had a decrease. All of these renal units had mild or no hydronephrosis at a median follow-up of 15 months, and none required intervention. The authors attributed these findings to the normal variability of hydronephrosis in early life. In contrast, all of the renal units that did require intervention had either [1] no change in hydronephrosis on the two postnatal sonograms or [2] obvious anatomic pathology that made serial imaging moot (eg, posterior urethral valves, ectopic ureterocele). Based on these results, the authors recommended that the initial postnatal sonogram be performed at age 7 to 10 days in newborns with a history of unilateral or mild bilateral prenatal hydronephrosis. They suggested obtaining an initial scan within the first day of life in cases of suspected oligohydramnios, urethral obstruction, multicystic renal dysplasia, bilateral moderate-to-severe hydronephrosis, or uncertainty of the prenatal diagnosis.

The Society for Fetal Urology proposed the following grading system for ultrasonographic findings of postnatal hydronephrosis based on the separation of the central renal complex and caliectasis [19,20]:

- Grade 0—intact central renal complex plus normal parenchyma
- Grade 1—slight central renal complex splitting plus normal parenchyma

- Grade 2—central renal complex splitting confined within renal border plus normal parenchyma
- Grade 3—wide splitting of central renal complex plus pelvis dilated outside renal border plus calices uniformly dilated plus normal parenchyma
- Grade 4—large dilated calices plus further dilation of renal penis plus thinning of parenchyma (ie, less than half that of the contralateral kidney). If bilateral hydronephrosis, then less than 4 mm is the cut off for parenchymal thinning.

The role of performing a VCUG in infants who have prenatal hydronephrosis and a normal postnatal ultrasonogram is controversial. With confirmed postnatal hydronephrosis, a VCUG is performed routinely to detect anomalies such as VUR and ectopic ureteroceles. Several studies have advocated deferring VCUG, with continued careful observation, in a subset of patients For example, Yerkes and colleagues evaluated 60 infants who had less than grade 2 unilateral or bilateral hydronephrosis seen on ultrasounds performed at 1 month of life [21]. Of these, 44 underwent VCUG as part of the early evaluation, and 16 were observed and kept on short-term antibiotic prophylaxis. Infants who had sonographic evidence of severe prenatal hydronephrosis, hydroureter, duplication, or small or echogenic kidney or bladder abnormalities were excluded from the study. VCUG was positive in 15% of the infants who had less than grade 2 hydronephrosis. Although this is significantly higher than the frequency of approximately 1% in normal children, none of the 16 infants in the observation group had deleterious renal events within the follow-up period of 6 months to 4.5 years. An obvious limitation to this study is the significantly smaller size of the observation group.

Neonates who have grade 3 to 4 hydronephrosis and suspected bilateral ureteropelvic or UVJ obstruction should undergo prompt diuretic renogram to evaluate differential renal function [22]. In the case of unilateral hydronephrosis and a normal contralateral kidney, functional renal studies may be delayed until the infant reaches 4 to 6 weeks of age. The two agents commonly used to evaluate for function and upper tract drainage estimates are technicium-99m-diethylene triamine pentaacetic acid ([^{99m}Tc] DTPA) and technetium-99m-mercaptoacetyltriglycine ([^{99m}Tc] MAG-3). MAG-3 is more expensive than DTPA but gives superior anatomic details on the images. When furosemide is administered during the renal scan, the study is referred to as a diuretic renogram. The well-tempered renogram is a standardized protocol that includes bladder catheter drainage and specific procedural details (eg, method of hydration and timing of furosemide administration) [23,24]. The half-life ($t_{1/2}$) is the rate of decline in radioactivity in the collecting system and is used to evaluate for obstruction:

- Nonobstructive drainage—0 to 10 minutes
- Indeterminate—10 to 20 minutes
- Obstruction—greater than 20 minutes [25]

Hydronephrosis: specific anomalies

Ureteropelvic junction obstruction

UPJ obstruction causes 44% to 65% cases of prenatal hydronephrosis and is the most common cause of severe hydronephrosis in a newborn without a dilated ureter or bladder [26]. UPJ obstruction, which is unilateral in 90% of cases, may result from an intrinsic narrowing at the junction between the ureter and renal pelvis or extrinsic compression by an accessory lower pole artery to the kidney [27]. A lesser degree of hydronephrosis may occur on the contralateral side. Controversy remains regarding the postnatal treatment of severe, unilateral, primary UPJ obstruction type, prenatally detected hydronephrosis. Palmer and colleagues reported the findings of a multicenter prospective randomized study from The Society for Fetal Urology on high-grade obstructive unilateral hydronephrosis [28]. They evaluated the benefits of pyeloplasty compared with untreated obstruction. The authors found that children younger than 6 months with good renal function and unilateral obstructive hydronephrosis had a better outcome with pyeloplasty than observation.

On the other side of the controversy are the advocates for nonoperative management of severe unilateral primary hydronephrosis, who propose that a high percentage of cases either resolve or improve. For example, Ulman and colleagues prospectively evaluated 104 newborns with severe (Society of Fetal Urology grades 3 and 4), unilateral, primary UPJ obstruction type hydronephrosis over a mean of 78 months [29]. All 23 infants (22%) who underwent pyeloplasty were younger than 18 months and had progressive hydronephrosis or reduction in differential renal function of greater than 10%. Differential renal function was greater in all kidneys postoperatively than it was before renal deterioration. Of those cases managed nonoperatively, hydronephrosis resolved in 69% and improved in 31%. Mean time to maximal improvement of hydronephrosis was 2.5 years. In 76% of cases managed nonoperatively, initial differential function was greater than 40%, and the final differential function was 47% on average.

One of the challenges in managing prenatal hydronephrosis is identifying the beginning of renal decompensation before the onset of permanent damage secondary to UPJ obstruction. Captopril renography may distinguish those patients with congenital UPJ obstruction type hydronephrosis who have renin–angiotensin system activation. Activation of this system signals the beginning of compensatory vasoactive response in the kidney. Minu and colleagues prospectively evaluated the results of captopril renography in 25 patients who had suspected unilateral congenital UPJ obstruction [30]. They found that renin–angiotensin system activation detected by captopril renography was positive in 8 of the 25 cases (32%) of unilateral hydronephrosis. All six patients who required surgery were retrospectively identified to have positive renin–angiotensin system activation. None of the patients with a nonactivated renin–angiotensin system required surgery. There may be a role for captopril renography for detecting compensatory mechanisms mediated by the renin–angiotensin system in obstructive uropathy.

Vesicoureteral reflux

There are no prenatal ultrasonographic signs specific for VUR. The usual finding with VUR is nonspecific hydronephrosis of variable degree. Overall, about 10% to 20% of patients who have prenatal hydronephrosis are diagnosed with neonatal VUR [31,32]. The degree of prenatal hydronephrosis is associated significantly with the incidence of reflux, but even severe hydronephrosis has only about a 30% to 35% incidence of reflux [32]. Thus, neither reflux nor its grade can be diagnosed accurately during the prenatal period. Megacystis–megaureter is the association of bilateral VUR, a massively dilated bladder, and bilateral hydroureteronephrosis. Most prenatal reflux occurs in boys, and it tends to be high-grade and bilateral [33]. Circumcision has been recommended for male neonates to decrease the risk of

urinary tract infections (UTIs), which may lead to further progression of renal scarring [33].

The American Urological Association has established the resolution rates and guidelines for the treatment of VUR based on grade and laterality [34]. The higher the grade and bilaterality of VUR is associated with reduced rates of resolution. The treatment options for VUR include observation with antibiotic suppression until radiographic confirmation of resolution of the reflux, endoscopic treatment with Deflux (Q-Med, Uppsala, Sweden), and ureteroneocystostomy.

Primary nonrefluxing megaureter

Nonrefluxing megaureter results from an aperistaltic segment of the distal ureter causing abnormal propulsion of urine. Ultrasonographic findings include a dilated ureter and renal pelvis with variable atrophy of the renal parenchyma. VCUG does not demonstrate VUR. Indications for a prompt well-tempered diuretic renogram include an abdominal mass, solitary kidney, or bilateral hydroureteronephrosis [22]. If none of these conditions are present, the diuretic renogram is postponed until 6 to 8 weeks of age. If differential renal function is at least 35% to 40%, the child may be managed nonoperatively with follow-up diuretic renograms every 3 to 6 months. Surgical correction involves excision of the aperistaltic segment, tapering of the ureter, and ureteral reimplantation.

The natural history of primary nonrefluxing megaureter is a tendency of gradual reduction in hydronephrosis over several years. McLellan and colleagues assessed clinical and ultrasonographic predictors of spontaneous resolution of prenatally diagnosed, primary nonrefluxing megaureter in 54 patients with a median follow-up period of 25.8 months [35]. Ten patients underwent surgical repair for severe hydroureteronephrosis. In 39 cases (72%) hydroureteronephrosis resolved; it persisted in five cases at 30 to 72 months of follow-up. Mean initial ureteral diameter in patients who had resolution was less than in those without resolution and in those who underwent surgery (0.8 versus 1.15 and 1.32 cm, respectively). Hydronephrosis grade at presentation was a significant predictor of resolution rate ($P = .03$). Grades 1 to 3 hydronephrosis resolved at a median age of 12.9, 23.9, and 34.6 months respectively. Patients who experienced resolution of grades 4 and 5 hydronephrosis did so at a median age of 48.5 months. Children who had primary nonrefluxing megaureter and grade 4 or 5 hydronephrosis or a retrovesical ureteral diameter of more than 1 cm were likely to require surgery. Shukla and colleagues confirmed the role for nonsurgical treatment of primary nonrefluxing megaureter with a mean follow-up period of 6.8 years [36]. Their study of 40 infants found a complete resolution rate of 52.5% at a mean of 2.9 years and improved or stable hydroureteronephrosis in 47.5% of the patients.

Ureterocele

A ureterocele is a cystic dilatation of the distal end of the ureter that causes obstruction. They may be ectopic (ie, extending through the bladder neck) or intravesical (ie, remaining entirely within the bladder). This condition is more common in girls and may be associated with a solitary collecting system or the upper pole of a completely duplicated collecting system. Prenatal ultrasonographic findings include either hydroureteronephrosis or upper pole hydronephrosis with a dilated ureter down to the bladder. An intravesical, cystic structure at the bladder base also is seen. Treatment options include endoscopic decompression of the ureterocele, upper pole heminephrectomy, nephrectomy, and full reconstruction with ureterocelectomy and ureteral reimplantation with or without upper tract surgery.

Endoscopic decompression has been advocated as the initial mode of treatment for ureteroceles, especially intravesical ureteroceles and those with a single system, and it has been shown to decrease the need for secondary surgery [37,38]. An obvious advantage of this treatment modality is that this is a minimally invasive technique. Several techniques have been used to endoscopically decompress (ie, incision or puncture) the ureterocele: electrocautery, stylet, cold knife, and potassium titanyl phosphate and holmium:YAG lasers [39–41]. Jankowski and Palmer recently showed that holmium:YAG laser can be used to successfully endoscopically puncture a ureterocele in the neonatal period [42].

One disadvantage of the endoscopic approach is that it may leave behind a nonfunctioning renal moiety associated with the ureterocele. Chertin and colleagues focused on the feasibility of endoscopic puncture of ureteroceles as a definitive procedure and the safety of leaving a nonfunctioning upper pole moiety in situ [43]. Of the 48 children in their series with a nonfunctioning or poorly functioning upper moiety, only 4%

required upper pole nephrectomy during a median follow-up period of 9 years because of recurrent UTIs. Four children, however, required secondary puncture, and two children ultimately required ureteral reimplantation.

The management of the extravesical ureterocele is controversial. Shekarriz compared the long-term results of these procedures with primary lower tract reconstruction in 106 patients who had extravesical ureteroceles [44]. In patients who had intravesical ureteroceles treated with endoscopic puncture, the overall reoperation rate was 22%, and it was 23% in those treated with endoscopic incision or puncture. In patients who had extravesical ureteroceles, the reoperation rate was 100% in the transurethral incision/puncture group, 41% in the group with an upper tract approach (partial or complete nephrectomy with partial ureterectomy or ureterostomy), and 0% in the complete reconstruction group (including ureterocelectomy or ureteral reconstruction with or without upper tract surgery). Although transurethral therapy seems to be effective in most patients who have intravesical ureteroceles, it is not definitive therapy in patients who have extravesical ureteroceles.

There may be a role for watchful waiting in select cases of prenatally detected ureteroceles. Direnna and colleagues retrospectively reviewed the outcomes of 10 patients with prenatally detected ureteroceles who had no evidence of ipsilateral lower pole moiety obstruction, high-grade (4 or 5) VUR, or bladder outlet obstruction [45]. No patient required surgical intervention over a median follow-up of 5 years. Han and colleagues prospectively identified 13 patients for nonoperative management who had ureteroceles associated with hydronephrosis or multicystic dysplasia [46]. Nine of the 13 patients required no surgical intervention. Three of the nine patients had either a nonfunctional upper pole moiety or a multicystic dysplastic kidney that involuted. Six had good function of the upper pole segments relative to the lower pole without high-grade obstruction on furosemide renography. Surgery was required for progressive obstruction in one patient and for breakthrough UTI in three patients. Furosemide renography may identify a subgroup of patients who are candidates for nonoperative management of ureteroceles. Ureteroceles with nonobstructed duplex systems have better preservation of renal function and a high rate of resolution of hydronephrosis and reflux.

Ureterovesical junction obstruction

UVJ obstruction typically is seen on prenatal ultrasonography as hydroureteronephrosis to the level of the bladder. The degree of hydroureteronephrosis is variable. The etiology includes an ectopic ureter and obstruction of a ureter positioned normally within the bladder. An ectopic ureter can be differentiated from a ureterocele by the presence of fetal upper pole hydroureteronephrosis in the absence of an intravesical cystic structure. The treatment involves resection of the obstructed ureteral segment and ureteroneocystostomy.

Posterior urethral valves

PUVs are the most common cause of bladder outlet obstruction in the newborn, with an incidence of approximately 1 in 5000 to 1 in 8000. The prenatal ultrasonographic presentation is hydronephrosis with oligohydramnios. Type 1 valves consist of leaflets that extend distally from either side of the verumontanum to the anterior urethral wall at the level of the urogenital diaphragm [47]. Type 2 valves, the most rare, extend from the proximal verumontanum toward the internal sphincter and bladder neck. Type 3 valves are composed of a diaphragm just distal to the verumontanum with a central perforation. Type 1 valves are more frequent (90%), whereas type 2 valves tend to cause more severe bladder and upper urinary tract obstruction. Prenatal sonographic findings are variable depending on the gestational age and severity of obstruction, but may include oligohydramnios, a dilated urinary bladder and posterior urethra (keyhole sign), bilateral hydronephrosis, and subcortical renal cyst formation [48]. The most important determinant of prognosis is the presence of a normal amount of amniotic fluid. Oligohydramnios or anhydramnios in association with bilateral hydronephrosis in the second trimester is nearly always fatal [48]. The early- to midterm prognosis for renal function, however, appears unchanged despite early prenatal detection [49,50]. In a study by Hutton and colleagues, second trimester findings that predicted a poor postnatal outcome were moderate or severe upper tract dilatation, defined as a renal anteroposterior diameter of 10 mm or greater, and increased echogenicity or cystic change in the renal parenchyma [49]. When these findings were present, 89% of patients were dead or had chronic renal failure at follow-up compared with 25% with mild upper tract dilatation in the second trimester or with bladder dilatation only [49].

The newborn may present with an abdominal mass, failure to thrive, urosepsis or urinary ascites. Work-up of suspected PUV consists of a renal and bladder sonogram to assess pelvic and calyceal dilatation and cortical echogenicity in addition to a VCUG to evaluate for vesicoureteral reflux. Initial treatment involves placement of a pediatric feeding tube to drain the bladder and management of possible electrolyte abnormalities. Surgical correction is done by means of transurethral valve ablation using a pediatric cystoscope and miniature Bugbee electrode. Other options include cutaneous vesicostomy, cutaneous pyelostomy/ureterostomy, percutaneous nephrostomy tube, and the Soberen-T temporary high diversion that entails a cutaneous ureterostomy and suturing of the distal ureter to the upper ureter just distal to the renal pelvis. Factors indicative of a good long-term prognosis include a serum creatinine level 1 month after urinary drainage of less than 0.8 to 1.0 mg/dL and the presence of a pop-off valve mechanism, such a unilateral VUR associated with a nonfunctioning kidney, a large bladder diverticulum, or urinary ascites. The pop-off valve allows the kidneys to develop without the deleterious effects of high pressure. Urinary ascites are caused by urine leakage out of the urinary tract after rupture of a kidney or bladder caused by high pressures [51]. Urine may leak directly into the peritoneal cavity, especially in females with a persistent urogenital sinus or cloacal malformation. In males with PUV, the usual site of leak is from the kidney into the retroperitoneum, and the urine then transudates across the thin peritoneum into the peritoneal cavity. In a study of 12 patients with urinary ascites with a 3- to 14-year follow-up, two patients died of causes related to pulmonary hypoplasia. Nine of 10 survivors had good renal function and urinary continence, and the remaining patient required dialysis [31]. Some patients may present with PUV in childhood manifested as UTIs and voiding dysfunction. In a retrospective study of 36 patients who presented after age 5 with PUV, renal function was impaired significantly compared with controls [52]. Mean serum creatinine levels were 1.03 mg/dL and 2.17 mg/dL in the early and late presenting cases, respectively ($P = .005$).

Megacystis–megaureter

Megacystis–megaureter is the association of bilateral VUR, a massively dilated bladder, and bilateral hydroureteronephrosis. Please refer to the section on vesicoureteral reflux.

Cystic renal disease

Multicystic dysplastic kidney

Prenatal ultrasonography is a sensitive tool to diagnose a multicystic dysplastic kidney (MCDK). The characteristic findings on ultrasound include multiple, variable-sized, noncommunicating cysts, no central large cyst, and minimal to no renal parenchyma [53,54]. In comparison, severe hydronephrosis has a medially positioned central cystic structure, with multiple dilated and relatively uniform-sized calyces located laterally and communicating with central cystic structure. It can be difficult to differentiate MCDK from severe hydronephrosis on prenatal ultrasonography, however, and postnatal study is needed to confirm the diagnosis. A multicystic dysplastic moiety may be associated with a duplicated collecting system, with the upper system being the more commonly affected moiety. Also, MCDK may be noted on postnatal physical examination, by an abdominal mass on routine examination, by impaired pulmonary function, or by impaired gastrointestinal function.

Postnatal radiographic imaging is essential to evaluating a child with either suspected or confirmed MCDK. A renal scan of a MCDK does not demonstrate function and is confirmatory of the diagnosis. Anomalies associated with the contralateral kidney include VUR and UPJ obstruction [22]. A VCUG is performed routinely because of the risk of VUR. In one series, 19 of 75 patients with MCDKs had contralateral reflux (26.4%), which was of grades 1 to 2 in nine patients [55]. After a median follow-up of 4.4 years spontaneous resolution was more common in patients with grades 1 and 2 (89%) versus grades 3 and 4 VUR (50%) ($P = .14$). Spontaneous resolution occurred in 68% of patients overall, with a mean time to resolution of 20.1 months. Interestingly, there were also no significant differences in contralateral renal length based on the presence or absence of contralateral VUR. There were also no significant differences detected in serum creatinine based on reflux status. These data suggest that contralateral reflux does not present a significant threat to renal growth and function in children with multicystic dysplastic kidney, and most cases of reflux resolve spontaneously. Patients who have MCDKs primarily can be followed up conservatively with routine ultrasonograms to monitor renal involution and malignancy development, and blood pressure measurements because of the risk hypertension development [22]. Involution occurs in approximately 25% of the cases, usually within about 14 months [56]. Nephrectomy usually is reserved for noninvoluting MCDKs, large MCDKs that interfere with respiratory or intestinal function in the neonatal period, or MCDKs with enlarging solid areas on follow-up ultrasonogram [57].

Autosomal recessive polycystic kidney disease (infantile polycystic kidney disease)

Autosomal recessive polycystic kidney disease (ARPKD) is another cystic condition identifiable on prenatal ultrasonography. The usually lethal condition in the newborn period, caused by pulmonary failure, is characterized by large, uniform, echogenic, renoform-shaped kidneys without visible cysts on ultrasonography. The sonographic appearance develops before 20 weeks of gestation. Oligohydramnios develop, which lead to the pulmonary failure and Potter's syndrome (ie, pulmonary hypoplasia, low-set ears, skeletal defects, and oligohydramnios). The multiple small cysts give a bright echogenicity on newborn ultrasonography. There is minimal disease-specific therapy to offer these newborns. The children with slower deterioration of renal function will develop pancreatic and hepatic cystic disease [58,59].

Other urologic conditions

Renal agenesis

Renal agenesis may be unilateral or bilateral. In the latter condition, the kidneys are not identifiable, and the bladder is not seen filling on prenatal ultrasonography in renal agenesis. Also, there is progressive decline of amniotic fluid volume after 16 to 18 weeks of gestation [60–62]. Potter's syndrome, a small thorax, and lying down adrenal relating to the linear appearance of the gland with its normal position are noted with renal agenesis [63].

Classic bladder and cloacal exstrophy

Classic bladder exstrophy and cloacal exstrophy arise within the first 8 weeks of gestation from abnormal mesodermal migration caused by an abnormal cloacal membrane overdevelopment during the development of the lower abdominal wall, and the anorectal and urogenital canals [64]. These conditions are diagnosed on prenatal ultrasonogram by an absence of bladder filling on serial examinations, a low-set umbilical cord, and external genitalia that appear abnormal. The affected newborn with classic bladder exstrophy is usually otherwise healthy with normal renal function and should undergo primary closure within 48 hours of birth [22]. In contrast, cloacal exstrophy is one of the most devastating congenital urologic abnormalities, and it often is associated with lower extremity abnormalities, myelodysplasia, and cardiac defects. Associated intestinal protrusion and omphalocele also may be detected prenatally. Parents with prenatally diagnosed exstrophy should be adequately counseled on the postnatal surgical interventions and long-term outcomes of these children.

Prune belly syndrome (Eagle-Barrett syndrome)

Prune belly syndrome may be caused by a transient congenital urethral membrane obstruction at 8 to 10 weeks of gestational age, followed by recanalization of the urethra and decompression of the urinary tract. The findings on prenatal ultrasonography, which typically are seen at 30 weeks of gestation, include bladder distention, hydroureters, and irregular, abdominal circumference dilation [65–67]. Although these findings suggest prune belly syndrome, the condition is difficult to differentiate from PUV or primary VUR. Classic newborn stigmata include a severely dilated bladder and upper urinary tract, bilateral intra-abdominal cryptorchidism, and abdominal flaccidity. The most important prognostic factor is the degree of renal impairment present. Severe renal dysplasia may lead to acute respiratory distress secondary to pulmonary hypoplasia or urosepsis, followed by neonatal mortality. Progression to renal failure is correlated strongly with bilateral abnormalities on renal ultrasonography or renography and a nadir serum creatinine greater than 0.7 mg/dL [68]. VCUG should be done promptly in infants with poor renal function, massive ureteral dilatation, a patent urachus, or high bladder residual volumes to delineate the urethral abnormalities, degree of bladder distention, extent of VUR, and the presence of urachal abnormalities. Surgical treatment of the dilated urinary tract remains controversial and should be tailored to the individual patient.

Urethral obstruction may be managed by urethrotomy, cutaneous vesicostomy, or progressive soft dilation of the urethra [68]. In the case of progressive azotemia, options for urinary tract decompression include bilateral open nephrostomies or early supravesical diversion by pyelostomy followed by total reconstruction [68]. Single-stage reconstruction consists of bilateral tapered ureteroneocystostomy, reduction cystoplasty, bilateral orchiopexy, and abdominoplasty. Denes and colleagues demonstrated that comprehensive surgical reconstruction can yield excellent long-term results [69]. Of 32 patients, 30 demonstrated stable or improved renal function at a mean follow-up of 5 years. No VUR was found postoperatively.

Myelomeningocele

Myelomeningocele is the most common congenital malformation of the central nervous system noted on prenatal ultrasonogram. Of these cases, 95% are diagnosed prenatally with a combination of ultrasonogram and maternal serum [alpha] fetoprotein. Spinal dysraphism is the most common cause of neurogenic bladder dysfunction in newborns. Fetal surgery to correct myelomeningocele theoretically could alter the damage sustained from constant exposure of the spinal cord to amniotic fluid. The results demonstrate a reduction in hindbrain herniation and the need for ventriculoperitoneal shunting but no significant impact on bladder function [70].

Genital abnormalities

In utero diagnosis of genital abnormalities, such as severe penile chordee or hypospadias, are diagnosed occasionally, while isolated epispadias is diagnosed rarely [71,72]. Physical examination should focus on the detection of gonads in the inguinal canal or scrotum and the identification of a possible uterus by means of a rectal examination. Of note, undescended testes in association with hypospadias also should prompt a work-up for ambiguous genitalia [73]. Initial laboratory studies should include a chromosomal analysis and serum studies for the byproducts of disordered steroid synthesis to exclude congenital virilizing adrenal hyperplasia. This condition may produce an enlarged clitoris and life-threatening adrenal crisis at 7 to 10 days of life.

Summary

Fetal urologic abnormalities encompass a broad spectrum of disease processes that present a challenge for the pediatric urologist and obstetrician. Knowledge about the specific conditions will help with prenatal counseling, determination of the need for therapeutic intervention in utero versus early delivery, and the postnatal evaluation and management of these conditions.

References

[1] Helin I, Per-Hakan P. Prenatal diagnosis of urinary tract abnormalities by ultrasound. Pediatrics 1986; 78:879.

[2] Cromie WJ, Lee K, Houde K, et al. Implications of prenatal ultrasound screening in the incidence of major genitourinary malformations. J Urol 2001;165: 1677.

[3] Siemens DR, Prouse KA, MacNeily AE, et al. Antenatal hydronephrosis: thresholds of renal pelvic diameter to predict insignificant postnatal pelvicalciectasis. Tech Urol 1998;4:198.

[4] Stocks A, Richards D, Frentzen B, et al. Correlation of renal pelvic anteroposterior diameter with outcome in infancy. J Urol 1996;155:1050.

[5] Docimo SG, Silver RI. Renal ultrasonography in newborns with prenatally detected hydronephrosis: why wait? J Urol 1997;157:1387.

[6] Ellsworth P, Sitnikova L. Impact of prenatal ultrasonography on the detection, evaluation, management and outcome of genitourinary anomalies. AUA Update Series 2005;24:235–52.

[7] Grignon A, Filion R, Filiatrault D, et al. Urinary tract dilatation in utero: classification and clinical application. Radiology 1986;160:645–7.

[8] Berhrman RE, Parer JT, deLannoy CW Jr. Placental growth and the formation of amniotic fluid. Nature 1967;214:678–80.

[9] Queenan JT, Thompson W, Whitfield C. Amniotic fluid volume in normal pregnancy. Am J Obstet Gynecol 1972;114:34–8.

[10] Potter EL. Normal and abnormal development of the kidney. Chicago: Year Book Medical 1972;209.

[11] Kaefer M, Peters CA, Retik AB, et al. Increased renal echogenicity: a sonographic sign for differentiating between obstructive and nonobstructive etiologies of in utero bladder distention. J Urol 1997;158:1026.

[12] Glick PL, Harrison MR, Mitchell SG, et al. Management of the fetus with congenital hydronephrosis II: prognostic criteria and selection for treatment. J Pediatr Surg 1985;20:376.

[13] Cromblethorme TM, Harrison MR, Golbus MS, et al. Fetal intervention in obstructive uropathy: prognostic indicators and efficacy of intervention. Am J Obstet Gynecol 1990;16:1239.

[14] Harrison MR, Filly RA, Parer JT, et al. Management of the fetus with a urinary tract malformation. JAMA 1981;246:635–9.

[15] Golbus MS, Harrison MR, Filly RA, et al. In utero treatment of urinary tract obstruction. Am J Obstet Gynecol 1982;142:383–8.

[16] Harrison MR, Nakayama DK, Noall RA, et al. Correction of congenital hydronephrosis in utero: II. Decompression reverses the effects of obstruction on the fetal lung and urinary tract. J Pediatr Surg 1982;17:965–74.

[17] Quintero RA, Hume R, Smith C, et al. Percutaneous fetal cystoscopy and endoscopic fulguration of posterior urethral valves. Am J Obstet Gynecol 1995; 172:206–9.

[18] Wiener JS, O'Hara SM. Optimal timing of initial postnatal ultrasonography in newborns with prenatal hydronephrosis. J Urol 2002;168:1826.

[19] Fernbach SK, Maizels M, Conway JJ. Ultrasound grading of hydronephrosis: introduction to the system used by the Society for Fetal Urology. Pediatr Radiol 1993;23:478.

[20] Maizels M, Reisman ME, Flom S, et al. Grading nephroureteral dilatation detected in the first year of life: correlation with obstruction. J Urol 1992; 148:609–14.

[21] Yerkes EB, Adams MC, Pope JC, et al. Does every patient with prenatal hydronephrosis need voiding cystourethrography? J Urol 1999;162:1218.

[22] Elder JS. Antenatal hydronephrosis: fetal and neonatal management. Pediatr Clin North Am 1997; 44:1299.

[23] Conway JJ. Well-tempered diuresis renography: its historical development, physiological and technical pitfalls and standardized technique protocol. Semin Nucl Med 1992;22:74–84.

[24] Society for Fetal Urology. The well-tempered diuretic renogram: a standard method to examine the asymptomatic neonate with hydronephrosis or hydroureteronephrosis. A report from combined meetings of the Society for Fetal Urology and members of the Pediatric Nuclear Medicine Council – The Society of Nuclear Medicine. J Nucl Med 1992;33:2047–51.

[25] Koff S, Thrall JH. Diagnosis of obstruction in experimental hydroureteronephrosis. Urology 1981;17: 570–7.

[26] Lim DJ, Park JY, Kim JH, et al. Clinical characteristics and outcome of hydronephrosis detected by prenatal ultrasonography. J Korean Med Sci 2003; 18:859–62.

[27] Livera LN, Brookfield DS, Egginton JA, et al. Antenatal ultrasonography to detect fetal renal abnormalities: a prospective screening programme. BMJ 1989;298:1421–3.

[28] Palmer LS, Maizels M, Cartwright PC, et al. Surgery versus observation for managing obstructive grade 3 to 4 unilateral hydronephrosis: a report from the society for fetal urology. J Urol 1998;159:222–8.

[29] Ulman I, Jayanthi VR, Koff SA. The long-term follow-up of newborns with severe unilateral hydronephrosis initially treated nonoperatively. J Urol 2000;164:1101.

[30] Minu B, Puri A, Tripathi M, et al. Prognostic significance of captopril renography for managing congenital unilateral hydronephrosis. J Urol 2002;168:2158.

[31] Elder JS. Editorial comment: importance of antenatal diagnosis of vesicoureteral reflux. J Urol 1992; 148:1750.

[32] Brophy MM, Austin PF, Yan Y, et al. Vesicoureteral reflux and clinical outcomes in infants with prenatally detected hydronephrosis. J Urol 2002;168:1716.

[33] Herndon CDA, McKenna PH, Kolon TF, et al. A multicenter outcomes analysis of patients with neonatal reflux presenting with prenatal hydronephrosis. J Urol 1999;162:1203.

[34] Elder JS, Peters CA, Arant Billy S Jr, et al. Pediatric vesicoureteral reflux guidelines panel summary report on the management of primary vesicoureteral reflux in children. J Urol 1997;157:1846–51.

[35] McLellan DL, Retik AB, Bauer SB, et al. Rate and predictors of spontaneous resolution of prenatally diagnosed primary nonrefluxing megaureter. J Urol 2002;168:2177.

[36] Shukla AR, Cooper J, Patel RP, et al. Prenatally detected primary megaureter: a role for extended follow-up. J Urol 2005;173:1353.

[37] Hagg MJ, Mourachov PV, Snyder HM, et al. The modern endoscopic approach to ureterocele. J Urol 2000;163:940–3.

[38] Blyth B, Passerini-Glazel G, Camuffo C, et al. Endoscopic incision of ureteroceles: intravesical versus ectopic. J Urol 1993;149:556–9.

[39] Marr L, Skoog SJ. Laser incision of ureterocele in the pediatric patient. J Urol 2002;167:280–2.

[40] Chertin B, Fridmans A, Hadas-Halpren I, et al. Endoscopic puncture of ureterocele as a minimally invasive and effective long-term procedure in children. Eur Urol 2001;39:332–6.

[41] Abrahamsson LO, Rosenkilde Olsen P, Mathiesen FR. Ureterocele in adults. A follow-up study of 28 adult patients treated with transurethral diathermy incision. Scand J Urol Nephrol 1981;15:239–42.

[42] Jankowski JT, Palmer JS. Holmium:yttrium-aluminum-garnet laser puncture of ureteroceles in the neonatal period. Urology 2006;68:179–81.

[43] Chertin B, Rabinowitz R, Pollack A, et al. Does prenatal diagnosis influence the morbidity associated with left in situ nonfunctioning or poorly functioning renal moiety after endoscopic puncture of ureterocele. J Urol 2005;173:1349.

[44] Shekarriz B, Upadhyay J, Fleming P, et al. Long-term outcome based on the initial surgical approach to ureterocele. J Urol 1999;162:1072.

[45] Direnna T, Leonar MP. Watchful waiting for prenatally detected ureteroceles. J Urol 2006;175:1493.

[46] Han MY, Gibbons MD, Belman AB, et al. Indications for nonoperative management of ureteroceles. J Urol 2005;174:1652.

[47] Krishnan A, de Souza A, Konijeti R, et al. The anatomy and embryology of posterior urethral valves. J Urol 2006;175:1214.

[48] Cendrom M, Elder JS. Perinatal Urology. In: Gillenwater JY, Grayhack JT, Howards SS, Mitchell ME, editors. Adult and Pediatric Urology. 4th edition. Philadelphia: Lippincott Williams & Wilkins; 2002. p. 2041–127.

[49] Hutton KA, Thomas DF, Davies BW. Prenatally detected posterior urethral valves: qualitative assessment of second trimester scans and prediction of outcome. J Urol 1997;158:1022.

[50] El-Ghoneimi A, Desgrippes A, Luton D, et al. Outcome of posterior urethral valves: to what extent is it improved by prenatal diagnosis? J Urol 1999;162:849.

[51] De Vries SH, Aart JK, Lilien MR, et al. Development of renal function after neonatal urinary ascites due to obstructive uropathy. J Urol 2002;168:675.

[52] Ziylan O, Tayfun O, Ander H, et al. The impact of late presentation of posterior urethral valves on bladder and renal function. J Urol 2006;175:1894.

[53] Sanders RC, Hartman DS. The sonographic distinction between neonatal multicystic kidney and hydronephrosis. Radiology 1984;151:621–5.

[54] Bearman SB, Hine PL, Sanders RC. Muticystic kidney: a sonographic pattern. Radiology 1976;118: 685–8.

[55] Miller DC, Rumohr JA, Dunn RL, et al. What is the fate of the refluxing contralateral kidney in children with multicystic dysplastic kidney? J Urol 2004;172: 1630.

[56] Ylinen E, Sirkku A, Ala-Houhala M, et al. Nephrectomy for multicystic dysplastic kidney: if and when? Urology 2004;63:768.

[57] Kuwertz-Broeking E, Brinkmann OA, von Lengerke HJ, et al. Unitlateral multicystic dysplastic kidney: experience in children. BJU Int 2004;93:338–92.

[58] Hussman KL, Friedwald JP, Gollub MJ, et al. Caroli's disease associated with infantile polycystic kidney disease: prenatal sonographic appearance. J Ultrasound Med 1991;10:235–7.

[59] Cole BR, Conley SB, Stapleton FB. Polycystic kidney disease n the first year of life. J Pediatr 1987; 111:693–9.

[60] Sherer DM, Thompson HO, Armstron B, et al. Prenatal sonographic diagnosis of unilateral fetal renal agenesis. J Clin Ultrasound 1990;18:648–52.

[61] Holmes LB. Prevalence, phenotypic heterogeneity and familial aspects of bilateral renal agenesis/dysgenesis. Prog Clin Biol Res 1989;305:1–11.

[62] Cardwell MS. Bilateral renal agenesis: clinical implications. South Med J 1988;81:327–8.

[63] Hoffman CK, Filly RA, Callen PW. The lying down adrenal sign: a sonographic indicator of renal

agenesis or ectopia in fetuses and neonates. J Ultrasound Med 1992;11:533–6.

[64] Marshall VF, Muecke C. Congenital abnormalities of the bladder. In: Baumbusch F, Schindler E, Schultheis TH, Vahlensieck W, editors. Handbuch de Urologie. New York: Springer-Verlag; 1968. p. 165.

[65] Christopher CR, Spinelli A, Severt D. Ultrasonic diagnosis of prune-belly syndrome. Obstet Gynecol 1982;59:391–4.

[66] Shih W, Greenbaum KD, Baro C. In utero sonogram in prune belly syndrome. Urology 1982;20:102–5.

[67] Bovicelli L, Rizzo N, Orsini LF, et al. Prenatal diagnosis of the prune belly syndrome. Clin Genet 1980;18:79–82.

[68] Strand WR. Initial management of complex pediatric disorders: prune belly syndrome, posterior urethral valves. Urol Clin North Am 2004;31:399.

[69] Denes FT, Arap MA, Giron AM, et al. Comprehensive surgical treatment of prune belly syndrome: 17 years' experience with 32 patients. Urology 2004;64:789.

[70] Holmes NM, Nguyen HT, Harrison MR, et al. Fetal intervention for myelomeningocele: effect on postnatal bladder function. J Urol 2001;166:2283.

[71] Mandell J, Bromley B, Peters CA, et al. Prenatal sonographic detection of genital malformations. J Urol 1995;153:1994–6.

[72] Benacerraf BR, Saltzman DH, Mandell J. Sonographic diagnosis of abnormal fetal genitalia. J Ultrasound Med 1989;8:613–7.

[73] Rajfer J, Walsh P. The incidence of intersexuality in patients with hypospadias and cryptorchidism. J Urol 1976;116:769.

ELSEVIER
SAUNDERS

Urol Clin N Am 34 (2007) 103–108

UROLOGIC
CLINICS
of North America

Index

Note: Page numbers of article titles are in **boldface** type.

Cystic renal disease, fetal, evaluation and
  management of, 97
    autosomal recessive polycystic kidney
      disease, 97
    multicystic dysplastic kidney, 97

Cystitis, acute, during pregnancy, 39

D

Denervation injuries, during vaginal delivery,
  13–14

Diagnostic imaging. *See* Radiology.

Dimethylsulfoxide, intravesical, for interstitial
  cystitis/painful bladder syndrome in pregnancy,
  63–64

Diversion. *See* Urinary diversion.

Drugs. *See* Pharmaceutical agents.

E

Eagle-Barrett syndrome, fetal, evaluation and
  management of, 98

Excretory urography, for suspected urolithiasis
  during pregnancy, 47

Expectant management, of urolithiasis during
  pregnancy, 48

Expulsive therapy, for urolithiasis during pregnancy,
  48–49

Exstrophy. *See* Bladder exstrophy *and* Cloacal
  exstrophy.

F

Fetal abnormalities, genitourinary, current diagnosis
  and management, **89–101**
    cystic renal disease, 97
    genital abnormalities, 98–99
    hydronephrosis, 89–97
      general considerations, 89–93
      specific anomalies, 93–97
    other urologic conditions, 97–98
      classic bladder and cloacal exstrophy, 98
      myelomenigocele, 98
      prune belly syndrome, 98
      renal agenesis, 97

Fistula, obstetric, 15

Fluoroquinolones, use during pregnancy, 29–30

Fluoroscopy, retrograde pyelogram, during
  pregnancy, 24

Functional changes, of lower urinary tract during
  pregnancy, **7–12**
  of upper urinary tract during pregnancy, **1–6**

G

General anesthesia. *See* Anesthesia.

Genital abnormalities, fetal, evaluation and
  management of, 98–99

Genitourinary changes, postpartum, **13–21**
    anal incontinence, 16–17
    denervation injury, 13–14
    elective primary cesarean delivery, 18
    genital tract trauma, 13
    obstetric fistula, 15
    operative injuries, 15
    pelvic floor muscle injury, 14
    pelvic organ prolapse, 17
    sexual function, 17–18
    urinary incontinence, 14–15
    urinary retention, 15–16

Glomerular filtration rate, during normal pregnancy,
  1–2

Glucose, renal handling of during normal pregnancy,
  4–5

H

Hemodynamics, renal, and glomerular filtration rate
  during normal pregnancy, 1–2
    mechanisms of alterations in, 2–3

Heparin, intravesical, for interstitial cystitis/painful
  bladder syndrome in pregnancy, 64–65

Hereditary conditions, interstitial cystitis/painful
  bladder syndrome, 65–66

Hydronephrosis, during pregnancy in patients with
  urinary diversion, 78
  fetal, 89–97
    general considerations for evaluation and
      management, 89–93
      diagnosis, 90–92
      fetal intervention, 92
      postnatal evaluation, 92–93
    specific anomalies, 93–97
      megacystitis-megaureter, 97
      posterior urethral valves, 96
      primary nonrefluxing megaureter, 94–95
      ureterocele, 95
      ureteropelvic junction obstruction, 93–94
      ureterovesical junction obstruction, 96
      vesicoureteral reflux, 94

Moving?

Make sure your subscription moves with you!

To notify us of your new address, find your **Clinics Account Number** (located on your mailing label above your name), and contact customer service at:

E-mail: elspcs@elsevier.com

800-654-2452 (subscribers in the U.S. & Canada)
407-345-4000 (subscribers outside of the U.S. & Canada)

Fax number: 407-363-9661

Elsevier Periodicals Customer Service
6277 Sea Harbor Drive
Orlando, FL 32887-4800

*To ensure uninterrupted delivery of your subscription, please notify us at least 4 weeks in advance of move.